BASIC CARDIOPULMONARY RESUSCITATION MANUAL

Edited by **Dr. José A. Morales González**

Basic Cardiopulmonary Resuscitation Manual

http://dx.doi.org/10.5772/56953
Edited by Dr. José A. Morales González

Authors

Cecilia Sánchez-Moreno, Evila Gayosso-Islas, José Antonio Morales-González, Reyna Cristina Jiménez-Sánchez, Mirandeli Bautista-Ávila, Ma. Luisa Sánchez-Padilla, Tomás Fregoso-Aguilar, Isaura Evelia Fuentes-Sánchez, Iván Villanueva-Becerril, Cristian Amaury Revoreda-Montes, Alejandro Chehue-Romero, Rocío Belém Mayorga-Ponce, Eva María Molina-Trinidad, Eufrosina Castillo-Arroyo, Jorge Gómez-Pedraza

Published by InTech

Janeza Trdine 9, 51000 Rijeka, Croatia

Publishing Process Manager Sandra Bakic
Typesetting InTech DTP Team
Cover InTech Design Team

Additional hard copies can be obtained from orders@intechopen.com

Basic Cardiopulmonary Resuscitation Manual,
Edited by Dr. José A. Morales González
p. cm.
ISBN 978-953-51-1201-3

For EU product safety concerns:
IN TECH d.o.o., Prolaz Marije Krucifikse Kozulić 3, 51000 Rijeka, Croatia,
info@intechopen.com or visit our website at intechopen.com.

Meet the editor

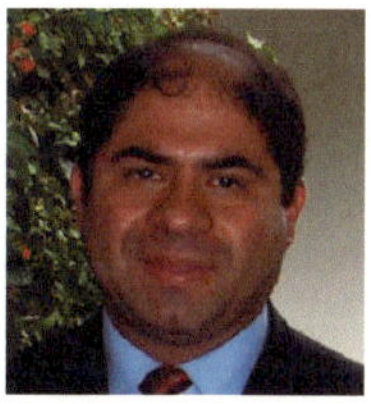

José Antonio Morales-González carried out his undergraduate rotating internship year at the Hospital de Jesus Public Welfare Institution (IAP) (1995), graduating as Surgeon Physician in 1997 from the Faculty of Higher Education (FES)-Iztacala National Autonomous University of Mexico (UNAM). He engaged in Doctoral studies in Biological Sciences (with a specialty in Cellular Biology) at the UNAM (1997–2001). Dr. Morales-Gonzalez has been awarded diverse recognitions: Hospital de Jesus IAP awards (1995 and 1996); Gustavo Baz Prada medal by the UNAM (1997); the Alfonso Caso medal for academic merit by the UNAM (2004); distinguished by the National System of Researchers (SNI) as National Researcher level 1 (2010-2016). He is the author of 45 internationally and nationally published articles. In addition to more than 200 citations to their publications. He is also editor and coordinator of 22 specialized books. Dr. Morales-González is a Full-time Titular Professor-Researcher Escuela Superior de Medicina, IPN

Contents

Authors

Evila Gayosso-Islas, M.Sc. Nursing

Undergraduate degree in Nursing and Obstetrics, National School of Nursing and Obstetrics (ENEO)-National Autonomous University of Mexico (UNAM). Mexico City, Mexico. Master of Nursing Sciences degree, Faculty of Nursing, Celaya Campus, University of Guanajuato, Mexico. Research Professor, Nursing Academic Area, Institute of Health Sciences (ICSa), Autonomous University of the State of Hidalgo (UAEH), Pachuca, Mexico.

Cecilia Sánchez-Moreno, M.Sc. Nursing

Undergraduate Degree in Nursing and Obstetrics, ENEO-UNAM, Mexico City, Mexico. Master degree in of Nursing Sciences, Faculty of Nursing, Celaya Campus, University of Guanajuato, Mexico. Research Professor, Nursing Academic Area, ICSa, UAEH, Pachuca, Mexico.

Reyna Cristina Jiménez Sánchez, M.Sc. Nursing

Undergraduate degree in Nursing and Obstetrics, ENEO-UNAM, Mexico City, Mexico. Master degree in Nursing Sciences, Faculty of Nursing, Celaya Campus, University of Guanajuato, Mexico. Research Professor, Nursing Academic Area, ICSa, UAEH, Pachuca, Mexico.

Ma. Luisa Sánchez- Padilla, M.Sc. Nursing

Undergraduate degree in Nursing and Obstetrics, ENEO-UNAM, Mexico City, Mexico. Master degree in Nursing Sciences, Celaya Campus, University of Guanajuato, Mexico. Master of Science degree in Educative Technology, UAEH, Pachuca, Mexico. Research Professor, Nursing Academic Area, ICSa, UAEH, Pachuca, Mexico.

Isaura Evelia Fuentes-Sánchez, B.Sc. Nursing

Undergraduate degree in Nursing, ICSa, UAEH, Pachuca, Mexico.

Cristian Amaury Revoreda-Montes, B.Sc. Nursing

Undergraduate degree in Nursing, ICSa, UAEH, Pachuca, Mexico. Educator in Diabetes with Multidisciplinary Focus, UAEH, Pachuca, Mexico. Consortium of Mexican Universities (CUMex) Scholarship, University of Applied Sciences, Münster, Germany.

Mirandeli Bautista-Ávila, Ph.D.

Undergraduate degree in Chemistry, UAEH, Pachuca, Mexico. Doctoral degree in Sciences, Complutense University, Madrid, Spain. Level 1 National Researcher. Title B Research Professor, Pharmacy Academic Area, ICSa, UAEH, Pachuca, Mexico.

Rocío Belém Mayorga-Ponce, M.Sc. Nursing

Undergraduate and Master degrees, Faculty of Nursing, Meritorious Autonomous University of Puebla (BUAP), Mexico. Research Professor, Nursing Academic Area, ICSa, UAEH, Pachuca, Mexico.

Eufrosina Castillo-Arroyo, M.Sc. Nursing

Undergraduate degree in Nursing, Autonomous University of the State of Morelos (UAEM), Cuernavaca, Mexico. Master degree in Nursing Sciences, Autonomous University of the State of Querétaro (UAQ), Mexico. Undergraduate degree in Law, Centro Hidalguense de Estudios Superiores, Pachuca, Mexico. Normative Coordinator of Nursing, Health Services in the State of Hidalgo, Pachuca, Mexico.

Tomás Fregoso-Aguilar, Ph.D.

Undergraduate degree in Biology, National School of the Biological Sciences-National Polytechnic Institute (ENCB-IPN), Mexico City, Mexico. Master degree in Physiological Sciences and Doctoral degree in Chemical-Biological Sciences, ENCB - IPN, Mexico City, Mexico. Title C Professor, Department of Physiology, ENCB-Zacatenco Campus, IPN, Mexico City, Mexico.

Iván Villanueva-Becerril, Ph.D.

Undergraduate degrees in Biology, IPN, Mexico City, Mexico with a Ph.D. degree in Chemo-Biological Sciences (specialized in Mammalian Physiology) and postdoctoral training in Physiological Regulation of Biological Rhythms. He currently is full-time professor of Human and Comparative Physiology at the National School of Biological Sciences In Mexico City. He is author of 10 original papers and a book chapter on physiological regulation and autonomic control.

Alejandro Chehue-Romero, M.Sc.

Undergraduate degree in Biology-Pharmacology-Chemistry, Faculty of Higher Studies (FES) Cuautitlán, UNAM, Mexico City, Mexico. Master of Sciences degree (Toxicology), ENCB, IPN, Mexico City, Mexico. Research Professor, Pharmacy Academic Area, ICSa, UAEH, Pachuca, Mexico.

Eva María Molina-Trinidad, Ph.D.

Undergraduate degree in Biology-Pharmacy-Chemistry, Faculty of Higher Studies (FES) Cuautitlán, UNAM, Mexico City, Mexico. Master degree in Pharmacy, Faculty of Chemistry, UNAM, Mexico City, Mexico. Doctoral degree in Chemistry, UNAM, Mexico City, Mexico. Level 1, National Researcher. Research Professor, Academic Area of Pharmacy, ICSa, UAEH, Pachuca, Mexico.

José Antonio Morales-González, Ph.D.

Undergraduate degree, Surgeon Physician, Faculty of Higher Studies, Iztacala Campus, UNAM, Mexico City, Mexico. Doctoral degree in Biological Sciences, Postgraduate degree in Biological Sciences, UNAM, Mexico City. Level 1 National Researcher.Escuela Superior de Medicina, Instituto Politécnico Nacional, México

Jorge Gómez-Pedraza, B.Sc. Nursing

Undergraduate degree in Nursing, ICSa, UAEH, Pachuca, Mexico. Research Professor, Nursing Academic Area, Institute of Health Sciences (ICSa), Autonomous University of the State of Hidalgo (UAEH), Pachuca, Mexico.

Preface

The purpose of this publication is to systematize the knowledge necessary to make Cardiopulmonary Resuscitation (CPR) or Cardiorespiratory Resuscitation (CRR) known to nursing health specialists, which translates as a set of temporary and internationally standardized maneuvers assigned to ensure the oxygenation of the vital organs when the blood circulation of an individual stops suddenly, independently of the cause of the Cardiorespiratory arrest (CRA). This knowledge is found correctly delimited in *The Basic Cardiopulmonary Resuscitation Manual,* which especially emphasizes the step-by-step methodology and techniques to follow for Cardiopulmonary Resuscitation (CPR). This is a basic work that cannot be overlooked by health care specialists, the society, and the public in general, because of the high probability that this situation will present at some moment in life. Thus, it is recommended to be prepared to help some person in an emergency situation. The manual is an excellent consultation work for health professionals.

In this manual, the chain of survival is considered within the CPR process. The chain of survival includes immediate activation of the Emergency medical system (EMS), early cardiopulmonary resuscitation (CPR), early Defibrillation (DF), and advanced care. This manual makes known the chronological order to follow prior to administering care to the victim with the purpose of establishing safety in the environment, type of patient, origin of the trauma, and the consideration of personnel qualified to respond to an emergency case of this nature. In addition to being a practical form of teaching, the manual makes known basic Cardiopulmonary resuscitation (CPR) in adults and CPR in pediatric patients and what leads to the learning of this technique. It also considers the updated information of American Heart Association (AHA) guidelines and the management of airways blocked by a foreign body. Similarly, in this manual the importance is depicted of the administration of the drugs utilized in CPR. Finally, it is of vital importance to consider the ethical aspects of basic CPR. Given that what is expressed in this work is fundamental for life, it has an intended purpose to and its objective is to make known the relevant information concerning the knowledge of CPR.

Authors

Chapter 1

Historical Antecedents

Over time, humans have sought ways to restore life to persons, aiding them with different techniques, employed by diverse cultures and religious-mythical-magical bases.

The reference most frequently alluded to and that which is considered the most ancient is that found in the Bible, in the Book of Kings (Kings II, 4:34–35), in which the manner is related in which Elijah placed his mouth, his eyes, and his hands on the mouth, eyes, and hands of a child who had just died and was able to return the child to life. Later, techniques were developed that at present appear strange to us, such as placing an unconscious person over a barrel and making it roll, or on a horse as it trots, with the intention of resuscitating the individual; these empirical techniques have inspired the basic principles of Cardiopulmonary resuscitation (CPR). During the World Wars and thanks to Anesthesiology, great advances were developed to revert Cardiopulmonary arrest (CPA), such as the exchange of bellows for bags (bag-valve- mask ventilator/resuscitator) to provide positive pressure and endotracheal intubation techniques.

Cardiopulmonary resuscitation has undergone important advances from the past century, and its sequence as we know it at present has led to an integrated process through the years, because at the beginning the techniques were known for permeabilizing the airways (the Esmarch-Heiberg maneuver), thoracic compressions thanks to Negovsky at the end of the 1940s and Kouwenhoven in 1960, and mouth-to-mouth resuscitation thanks to Elan in 1958. However, it was Peter Safar who integrated this knowledge and initiated what we now know as Cardio-pulmonary resuscitation (CPR).

Peter Safar is known as the father of modern CPR, because he demonstrated that with simply raising the chin the airway would be permeabilized, and integrating the researches of Elan and Kouwenhoven, he created what we know as the ABCs of cardiopulmonary resuscitation. He also established blood irrigation of the brain and clarified that even when cardiac activity could be established, if this were not done rapidly there is a high risk of brain damage. Likewise, he proposed of ambulances in which adequate pre-hospital care could be provided during the transport of the patient and that victims could arrive under conditions for their intra-hospitalary care. Safar thought that the success of these techniques resided in teaching these to as many people as possible.

The beginnings of the American Heart Association (AHA) were in 1915 in New York City, when some physicians and social workers met to work on the prevention and diminution of cardiac diseases. Due to this effort, professionals from other cities met to continue actions and researches, which gave rise to the creation of the AHA in 1924, made up of six physicians.

Through the years, the association has become strengthened with the drives for contributions that it conducts and with the scientific investigations of numerous professionals, which has favored the creation of protocols and recommendations that are followed nearly worldwide in relation to CPR and cardiac disease. The American Heart Association is concerned with exerting an impact on the social conscience in terms of cardiovascular risks, fortifying learning, no matter the age, integrating children into their programs.

The AHA maintains their programs and protocols updated, with the most recent contribution being the 2010 American Heart Association Guidelines for Cardiopulmonary Resuscitation, with the novelty of the implementation element algorithm Locally Enabled, Globally Optimized (LEGO) steps for resuscitators (see Chapter 5).

Chapter 2

Chain of Survival

As in all processes, success is determined by the correct execution of their steps. In Cardiopulmonary resuscitation (CPR), the sequence of the steps is decisive, does not permit delay, and survival of the victim can only be guaranteed if it is performed immediately, in orderly fashion, and correctly.

The American Heart Association (AHA) published a sequence of decisive interventions for acting in the face of Cardiopulmonary arrest (CPA); this is known as the chain of survival. This chain possesses the following critical links presented in sequence (Figure 2-1).

- Immediate activation of the Emergency medical system (EMS).
- Early Cardiopulmonary resuscitation (CPR).
- Early Defibrillation (DF).
- Early advanced care.

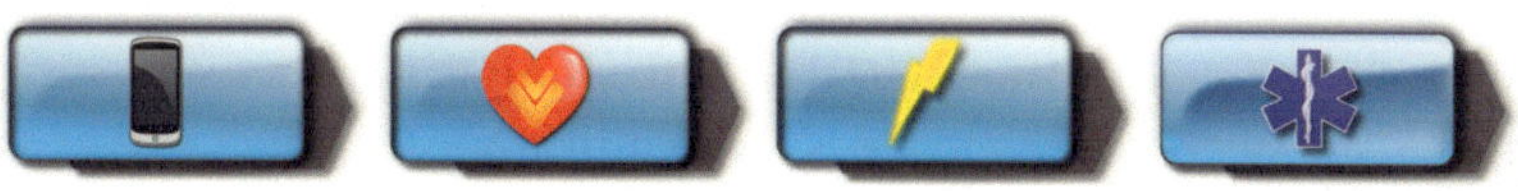

Figure 2-1. Chain of survival. Series of steps to follow in any accident, from arrival on the scene of the accident until trained personnel present.

Chain of survival in adults

First link: Activation of the emergency medical system

This consists of the timely identification of the situation from the level of consciousness of the patient, as well as the timely activation of the EMS. Timely identification of the signs of Respiratory arrest (RA) or Cardiopulmonary arrest (CA) guarantees immediate and adequate treatment of the victim.

Second link: Early cardiopulmonary resuscitation

The AHA emphasizes the importance of CPR for the treatment of cardiopulmonary arrest, especially thoracic compressions, as the best measure that can be implemented in this case.

The resuscitator, applying CPR maneuvers, can gain time for activating the EMS, if the resuscitator is found alone.

CPR maneuvers, especially thoracic compressions, increase in great measure the survival of victims affected by CA, in addition to these being easy-to-apply maneuvers, by specialized health care personnel as well as by the public in general.

Third link: Early defibrillation

Cardiac arrest (CA) can be caused by an abnormal heart rhythm, known as ventricular fibrillation, which is a rapid and irregular ventricular rhythm that leads to the complete loss of cardiac contractibility, lack of pumping, and death if it does not act. Rapid intervention is decisive for reverting this state; defibrillation is considered to be timely when it takes place within the first 5 minutes of the cardiac event.

The AHA proposes the placement of Automatic external defibrillators (AED) in public sites and of medical care vehicles to diminish intervention times.

Fourth link: Early advanced care

The previous steps are carried out by persons who have first contact with the victim and who can identify the signs of Cardiopulmonary arrest (CPA) and who can perform CPR and even use an AED. On arrival of the specialized services, the responsibility is transferred to these individuals to stabilize and transport the victim utilizing mechanical devices such as the Bag-valve ventilation mask (BVM), endotracheal cannulas, or invasive methods, such as endotracheal intubation, peripheral venous accesses for solutions and/or drugs, and oxygen therapy.

These links depend strictly on each other; in order to increase survival, all of the links should be evaluated and if one is omitted or not performed adequately, hope for life diminishes.

Pediatric chain of survival

There is a variant in the survival chain with recommendations for pediatric patients; the links are very similar, but emphasis is placed on Cardiopulmonary arrest (CPA) and its prevention (Figure 2-2).

- Prevention of Cardiopulmonary arrest (CPA).
- Early Cardiopulmonary resuscitation (CPR).
- Activation of the Emergency medical system (EMS).
- Early advanced care.
- Post-resuscitation care.

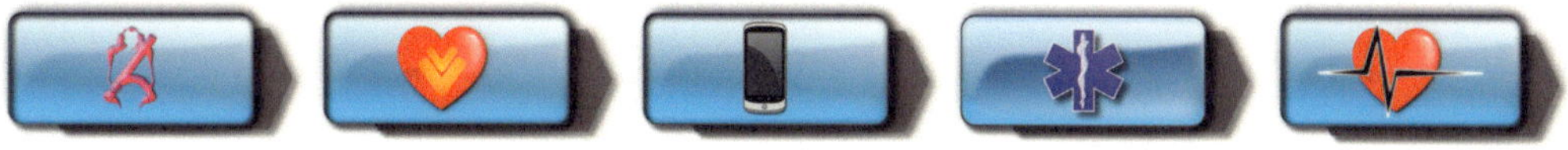

Figure 2-2. Pediatric chain of survival. Series of steps to follow, from arrival at the scene of the accident until trained personnel present.

Chain of survival (2010 update)

According to the description of the chain of survival published in the 2010 AHA Guidelines, a new link is integrated that makes reference to post-resuscitation care (Figure 2-3), thought to improve the survival of victims after cardiac and respiratory function is reestablished on admittance to the hospital unit. A multidisciplinary intervention is proposed to diminish possible complications.

The fundamental objectives are the following:

Provide cardiorespiratory support, with emphasis on perfusion of the organs, especially the brain.

Facilitate admittance to the Emergency room (ER) and the specialized Intensive care unit (ICU).

Assess and diagnose the factors that could give rise to Cardiorespiratory arrest (CRA) for the prevention of its reappearance.

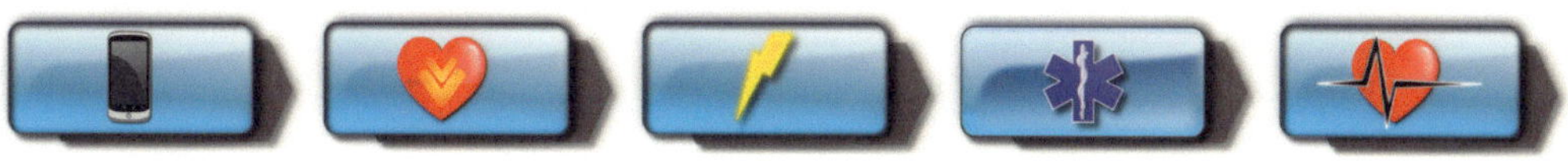

Figure 2-3. Chain of survival that includes the fifth link related with post-resuscitation care, proposed by the 2010 Guidelines of the American Heart Association (AHA). The chain has as its initial point the immediate care for Cardiorespiratory arrest (CRA).

Chapter 3

Initial Steps

Within pre-hospitalary care, there is a check list that comprises the steps prior to hospital care for the victim. These steps are focused on establishing safety in the environment, determining the number of victims, identifying the mechanism originating the trauma or the disease, as well as identifying the need for qualified personnel.

Assessing potential risks

As the first step, the risks should be assessed at the scene of the accident; ensure that there are no potential risks for the assistants, in the case of the latter being first responders, who in no way can serve by submitting themselves to a dangerous situation even if a potential risk is observed for the victim; the assistant should not approach any dangerous scene unless trained to do so; remember, first comes the safety of the assistant him/herself, above that of the victim (Figure 3-1).

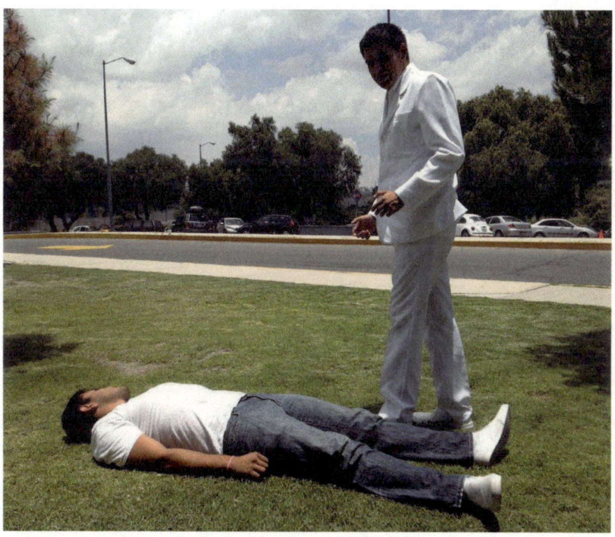

Figure 3-1. Initial evaluation in search of potential risks or mechanisms of injury.

There are three elements in this first evaluation step:

What is happening? and Under which conditions is this taking place?: Usually someone who is not accustomed to this situation can allow him/herself to be influenced by the victim's condition without observing the environment and the risks that accompany it.

What can be expected of the situation?: The different scenarios that are involved in an emergency condition can evolve into out-of-control situations; if the situation is analyzed adequately, occurrences that put the life of the responder and that of the victim in danger can be prevented.

The mechanics of the injury: On assessing the scene, we can find elements that are suspected to be involved in the victim's condition; for example, we might be able to see a person lying on the floor near a staircase, which would lead us to suspect a fall from above the level of the person's own height; an automobile accident in which the driver's windshield, or an unconscious person near high tension electrical cables. These elements permit us to emit a diagnosis of suspicion and to implement actions according to the victim's possible injuries.

Finally, it is useful to ask certain checklist questions, such as the following: Is the scene safe? Is there some potential risk? Are there more victims?

Assessing the state of consciousness

The second step is to evaluate the victim's state of consciousness by means of the victim's response. This can be assessed in a simple manner, asking some questions while grasping the shoulders of the victim and asking him/her the following: Are you all right? Can you talk? Can you hear me? and slightly shaking the victim by the shoulders (Figure 3-2).

We now find ourselves with two definitive variants: the victim responds, or the victim does not respond. In the first case, this would be very useful because we are able to consider a victim who responds to be alert; consequently, we would be able to establish a diagnosis regarding the victim's state by means of questioning and physical exploration.

Recall that a victim can be apparently unconscious due to multiple causes, such as trauma, drug use, alcohol use, or illness. Correct diagnosis will serve to determine the origin of the victim's state and the adequate treatment.

When the victim does not respond, the victim is automatically declared to be unconscious, even when the causes have not yet been determined; a measure to be enacted should be activation of the Emergency medical system (EMS). Remember that this activation can be different depending on the region or the country, and one should be prepared to know the specific emergency number that should be dialed.

If there are witnesses, these can be useful; one of these witnesses can be asked to activate the EMS and to request an ambulance. This should be requested specifically and imperatively, for example: **You, call an ambulance! You, dial 911 and ask for an ambulance!** You should be direct with a certain person in particular; if we make an open request, it is very probable that we will be ignored; it is difficult for persons to accept intervening in an emergency situation, perhaps due to their fearing involvement and being assigned responsibility for their action.

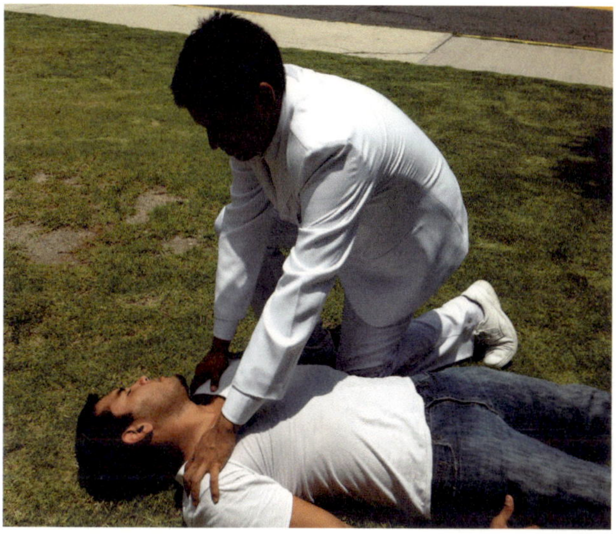

Figure 3-2. Evaluating the state of consciousness permits discarding situations that put life in danger in an immediate manner.

Once these steps are completed, we can begin to conduct the primary evaluation, which centers on detecting the emergency situations that place the life of the victim in immediate danger, in the following sequence of importance (A-B-C):

a. Airway.

b. Breathing.

c. Circulation.

Chapter 4

Basic Cardiopulmonary Resuscitation in Adults

Basic Cardiopulmonary resuscitation (CPR) is defined as an emergency procedure that allows the reestablishment of the respiratory and cardiac function of an individual who presents Cardiorespiratory arrest (CRA), without attending to, in the first instance, the causes that led to this, and counting on only our hands and our senses to perform the care.

The A-B-C of Cardiopulmonary resuscitation (CPR)

Initially, this consists of three elements, which are described as "A" (*Airway*), which corresponds to the maneuvers directed toward permeabilizing the airways, "B" (*Breathing*), in which ventilatory support actions are performed, and "C" (*Circulation*), focused on the effect of thoracic compressions.

The A-B-C denomination corresponds to the first letter of each of the components in English, as well as to the first three letters of the alphabet mnemotechnically, alluding to the sequence and the order of the steps.

A. Airway management

To achieve airway permeabilization, it is important to perform the technique adequately, thus ensuring successful artificial ventilation. Remember that during unconsciousness, muscle relaxation presents, and that due to incorrect positioning of the neck or of the internal structures of the neck itself, these can generate obstruction. This situation is quite determinant, but at the same time quite easy to correct, that it would ensure, with a sole change in the position of the victim's neck, that the latter's life can be saved,

Neck extension maneuver

Formerly, hyperextension of the neck would be requested for airway permeabilization, but this extension was identified as excessive in that in itself it could obstruct the airway, as takes place with tube that is flexed too much and becomes bent; similarly, the spinal column can be damaged, and currently it is recommended only to extend/tilt the neck.

Steps to permeabilize the airway:

1. Place a hand on the victim's forehead.
2. Place the index finger of the other hand on the victim's chin, being especially careful to support ourselves on the bony part.

3. Apply pressure backward with the hand situated on the forehead at the same time pulling up with the hand situated on the chin (Figure 4-1).

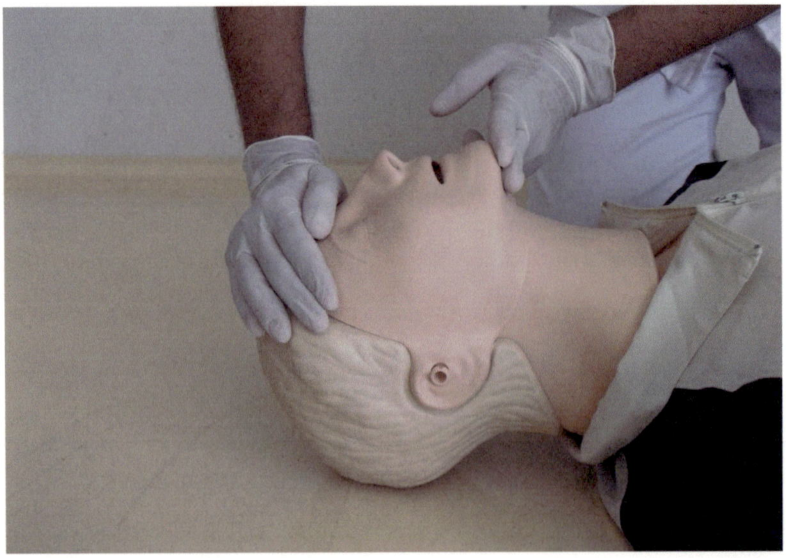

Figure 4-1. Correct maneuver for carrying out neck extension/tilting and in this way permeabilizing the airway. At present, only neck extension is recommended for permeabilizing the airway instead of hyperextension, which in itself can cause anatomical occlusion.

Jaw traction maneuver

This is a maneuver that is similarly useful for permeabilizing the airway.

1. Take the lower jaw of the victim in both hands at an angle.
2. Exert traction and at the same time turn the victim's head up, avoiding excessive pulling of the neck.
3. With the thumb, pull downward on the corner of the lips to permit ventilation (Figure 4-2).

Modified triple maneuver

This maneuver is recommended when some injury is suspected in some segment of the spinal column.

1. The hands are placed on both sides of the victim's head.
2. Take hold of the lower jaw at an angle.
3. Tilt the jaw downward.

This is also known as the E–C maneuver due to the way of placing the fingers on the jaw and the face (Figure 4-2).

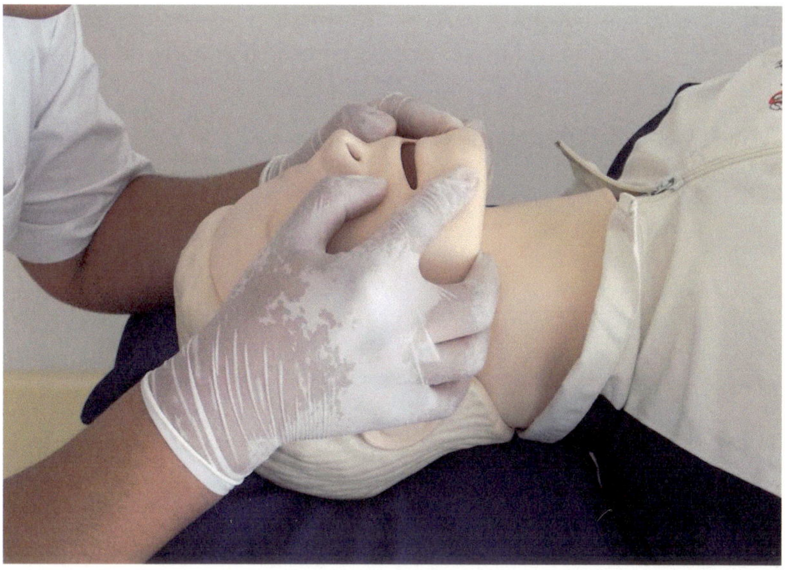

Figure 4-2. The modified triple maneuver, which guarantees the neutral position of the head and that is useful in the case of cervical injury. Modified triple maneuver or the E-C maneuver, so-called because of the position that the fingers take on placing these on the chin and the face, as shown in the image.

This maneuver can be complicated to maintain. Thus, the presence of another assistant is recommended.

B. Breathing

As a priority, it is necessary to reestablish spontaneous breathing in the victim and to evaluate the frequency and intensity of this function at another time.

In the case of breathing not being present or only an effort in the form of panting or gasping for breath, artificial ventilation should be initiated. Ventilation can be provided with the mouth-to-mouth resuscitation technique, even when this may not be very acceptable due to the conditions that the victim can present (hemorrhage or secretions). Currently, the choice is made in terms of how great the risk is of disease contagion by contact with secretions; thus, it is recommended whenever possible to utilize devices that can function as a barrier between the victim and the assistant to diminish the risk. Some of these devices are easy to use and those such as Bag-valve masks (BVM) do not require specific training.

As an important datum during mouth-to-mouth resuscitation, it should be considered that there is a concentration of approximately 21% of oxygen in the air. Therefore, the air that we expire contains a lesser amount.

To know whether the victim requires artificial ventilation, we must prove that the victim is not breathing. For this, we will employ a technique that although it is not indicated for Locally Enabled, Globally optimized (LEGO) resuscitators, according to the 2010 AHA Guidelines, it continues to be valid for health professionals and for trained personnel for identifying and differentiating between Cardiac arrest (CA) and Respiratory arrest (RA). This is known as the **S**ee **H**ear **F**eel (**SHF**) technique and it is performed during 5 or more than 10 seconds (Figure 4-3).

- **S**ee the thoracic expansion during the breathing.
- **H**ear the breathing.
- **F**eel the breath.

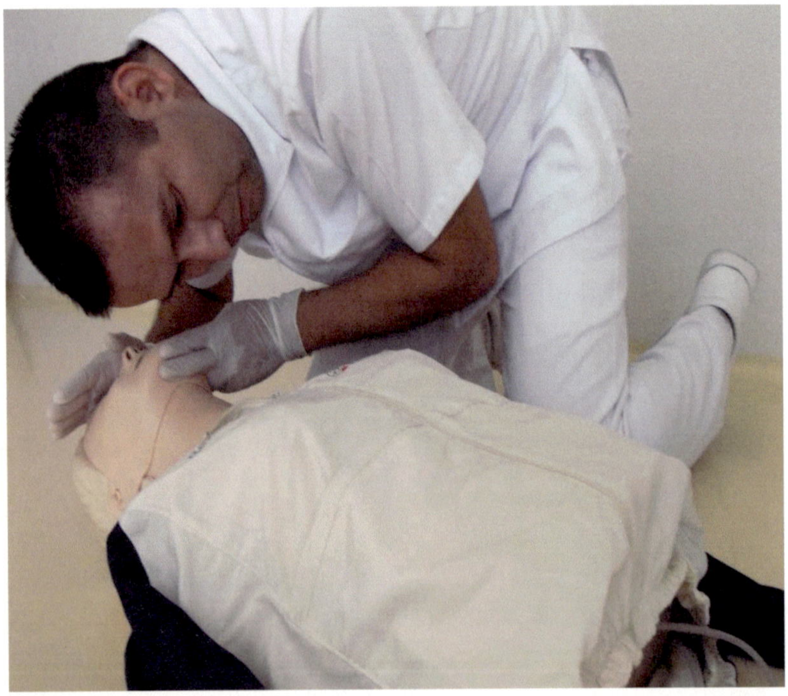

Figure 4-3. For identifying breathing, the cheek should be placed on the face of the victim; only thus can the air of the breathing be perceived and heard, in addition to appreciating the expansion of the thorax. If nothing is observed or perceived, one may think of a respiratory arrest or an airway obstruction.

If breathing is not perceived, two ventilations are administered, each with a duration of 1 second (Figure 4-4); the mouth-to-mouth technique should link the following conditions to be considered effective:

- There should be a perfect seal with the mouth of the victim.
- The nose should be occluded with the thumbs and index fingers (Figure 4-5).
- The ventilation should last one second.
- The insufflated air should correspond to a normal breath.
- During ventilation, the chest should be raised.

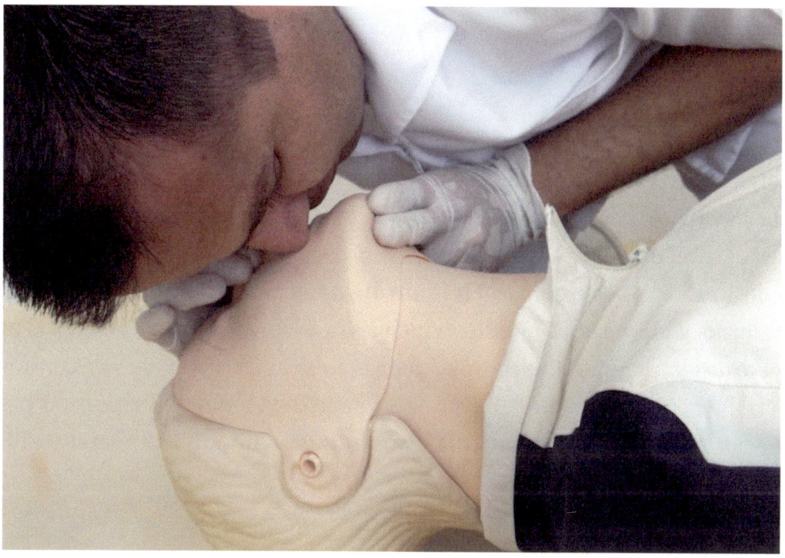

Figure 4-4. Correct way of carrying out the ventilations. The objective of the ventilations is to compensate for the lack of oxygen. The air that is insufflated contains approximately 16% of oxygen, but this can be sufficient for maintaining the victim.

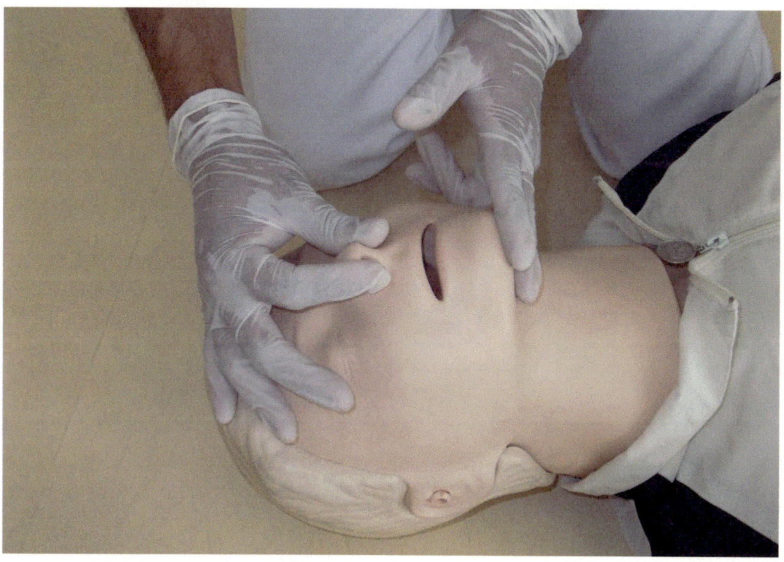

Figure 4-5. The image demonstrated the correct way to occlude the nose and to extend the neck of the victim. For mouth-to-mouth breathing to be effective it should join together certain conditions; an incorrect technique does not ensure the effectiveness of the procedure.

Excessive or excessively rapid ventilation, with incorrect neck extension, can direct the air to the stomach, consequently giving rise to what is known as gastric distension. In addition to these types of ventilation being ineffective, they can present vomiting (emesis) and the risk of bronchoaspiration.

C. Circulation

After administering the two ventilations, the carotid artery pulse should be assessed at a time between 5 and 10 seconds. This artery is useful thanks to its caliber and its proximity to the heart; it is localized and palpated easily, by solely placing the index and the middle fingers on the bony part of the chin (Figure 4-6), sliding the fingers until finding the cridoid cartilage (the Adam's apple, as it is known in males) (Figure 4-7), and finally sliding these to one side until finding the sternocleidomastoid muscle, which is that which forms a "V" in the neck (Figure 4-8). As a precaution, palpate the pulse of the same side that you are on; contrariwise, you could lean on the neck and occlude the air or damage the victim. If the pulse is palpated, it is only found prior to RA. Remember that RA can present without the necessity of CA, but not contrariwise.

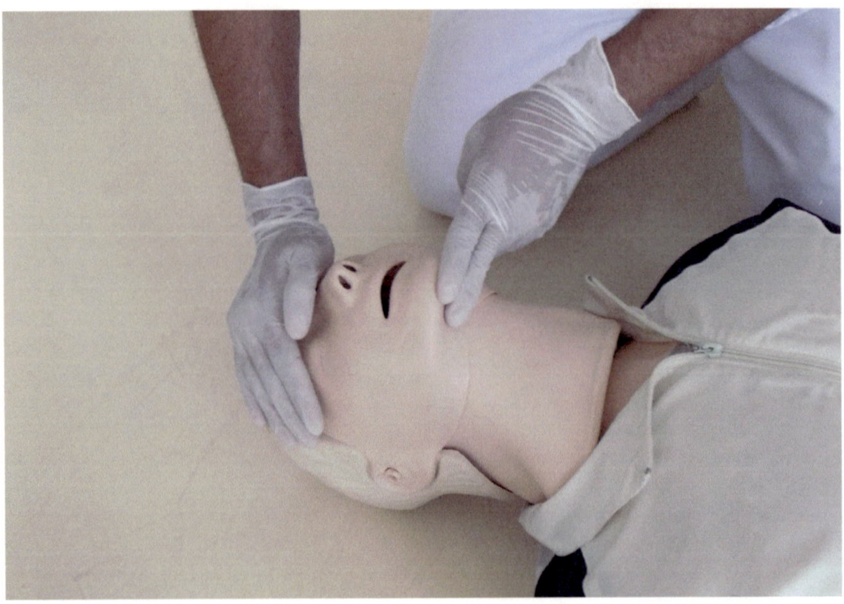

Figure 4-6. The image illustrates the correct way to place the fingers on the victim's chin. Place the thumbs and index fingers on the chin, thus preventing exerting pressure on the larynx and obstructing the passage of air accidentally.

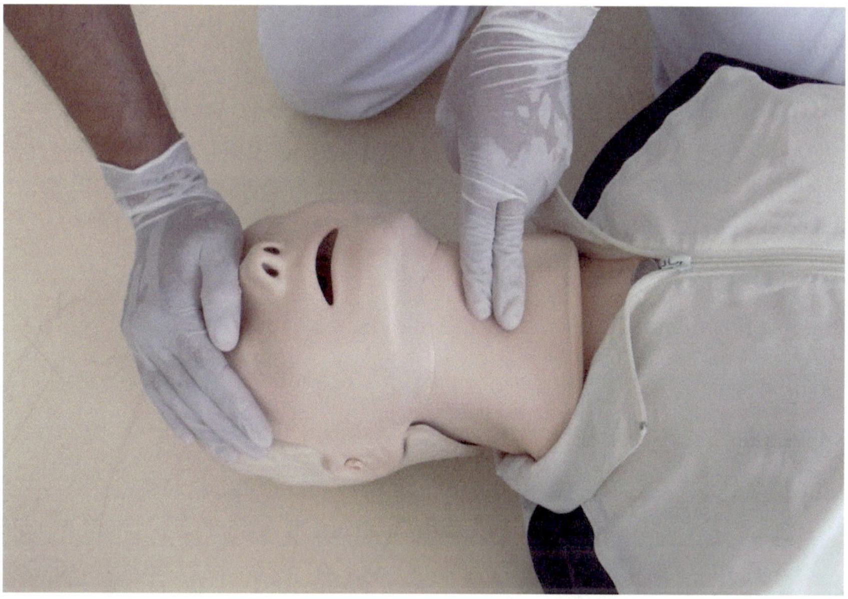

Figure 4-7. Slide the fingers naturally until touching the cricoid cartilage, being careful not to exert pressure during the movement.

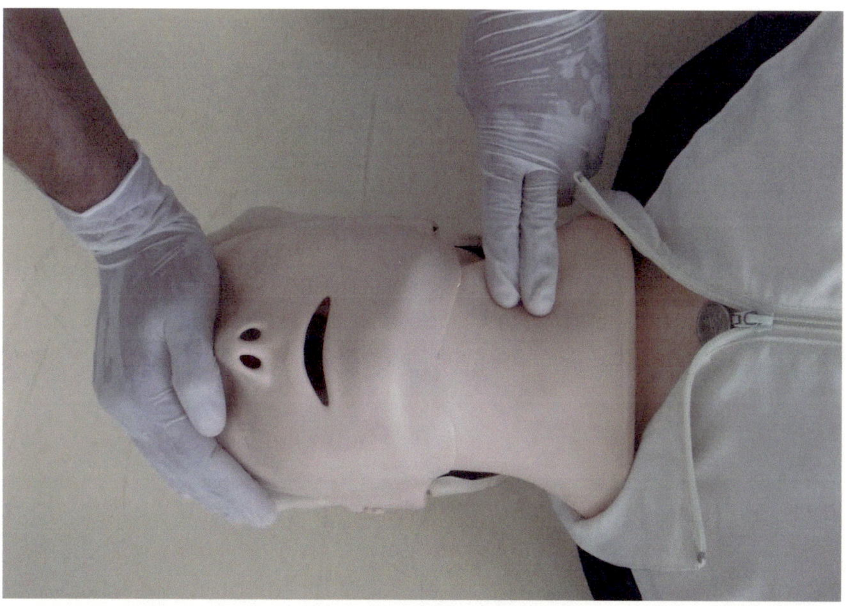

Figure 4-8. Even without much experience, the cardiac pulse is easy to palpate due to its thick caliber. In addition, it is chosen for its proximity to the heart. The thumbs and fingers are slid sideways until reaching the sternocleidomastoid muscle and finding the pulse.

If there is a doubt about the victim's pulse or if it is difficult to perceive it, do not lose time: begin thoracic compressions. Initiating CPR maneuvers even when the victim may not need them is less harmful than needing them, not proving them, and losing valuable time. The thoracic compressions should be applied at a rhythm of 30 compressions for every 2 ventilations at a rhythm of at least 100 ventilations per minute. Formerly this was suggested as approximately 100 per minute. Thoracic compressions should comply with the following conditions to be effective:

- Slide the fingers along the rib cage (Figure 4-9).
- Two fingers of the hands should be placed above the xiphoid appendix (Figure 4-10).
- Place one hand over the other above the previously mentioned point (Figure 4-11).
- The arms should be kept straight.
- The compression is performed with the weight of the torso of the assistant.
- The back should be straight (Figure 4-12).
- The glance of the assistant will fall naturally on the victim's other side (Figure 4-13).
- The thorax should be compressed at least 5 cm or 2 inches.
- After each compression, the thorax is allowed to expand again.

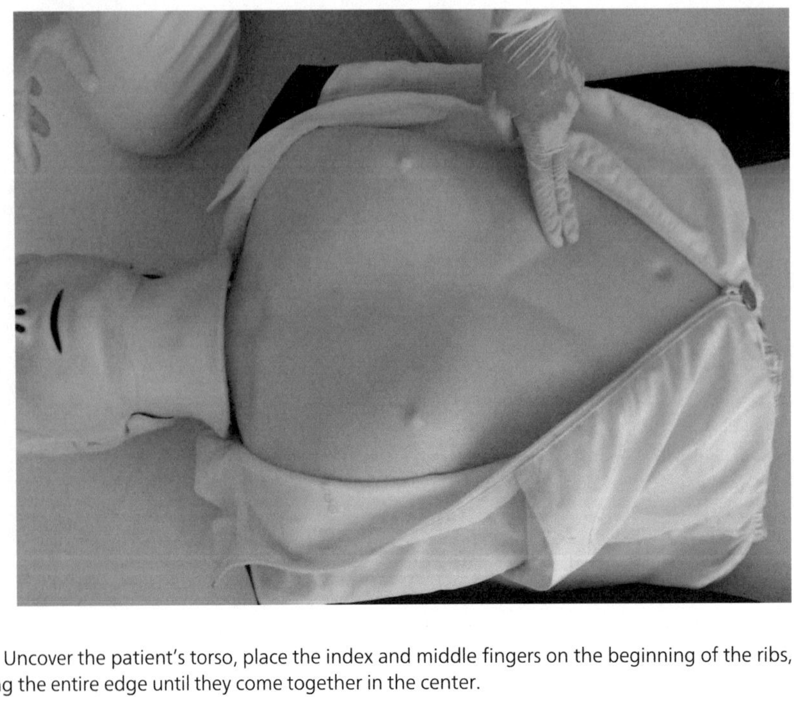

Figure 4-9. Uncover the patient's torso, place the index and middle fingers on the beginning of the ribs, and slide the fingers along the entire edge until they come together in the center.

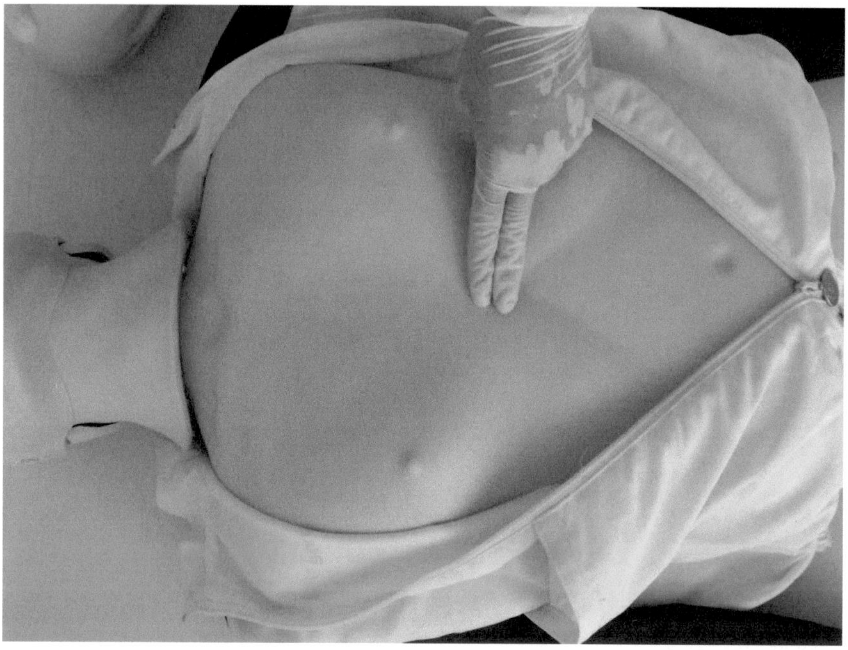

Figure 4-10. Once the xiphoid appendix is identified, place the index and middle fingers as depicted in the image.

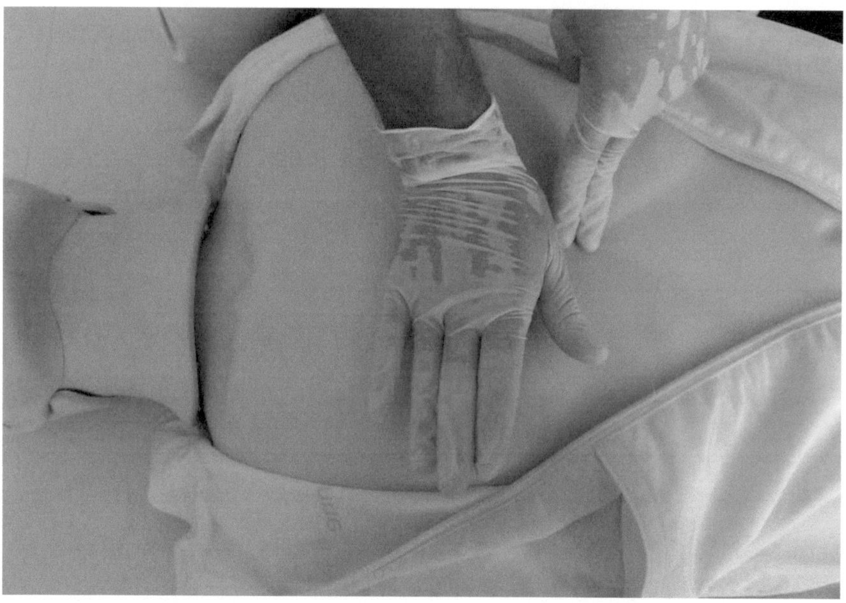

Figure 4-11. The correct way of placing the hands on the chest, to concentrate force in the center. The hand is placed above the index and middle fingers as observe in the image, this being the correct application site of the thoracic compressions.

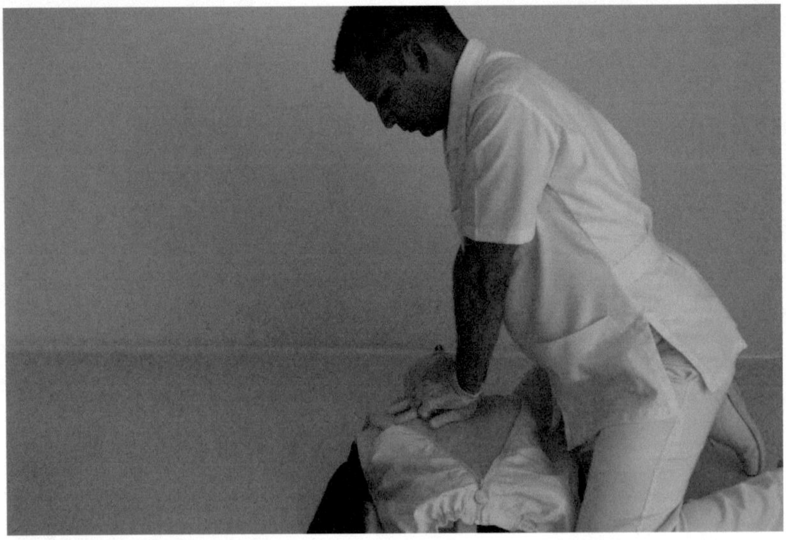

Figure 4-12. Identifying the site of application, place one hand over the other and initiate the thoracic compressions, taking care that the force is generated with the weight of the trunk to render these more effective and less tiring, as can be observed in the image.

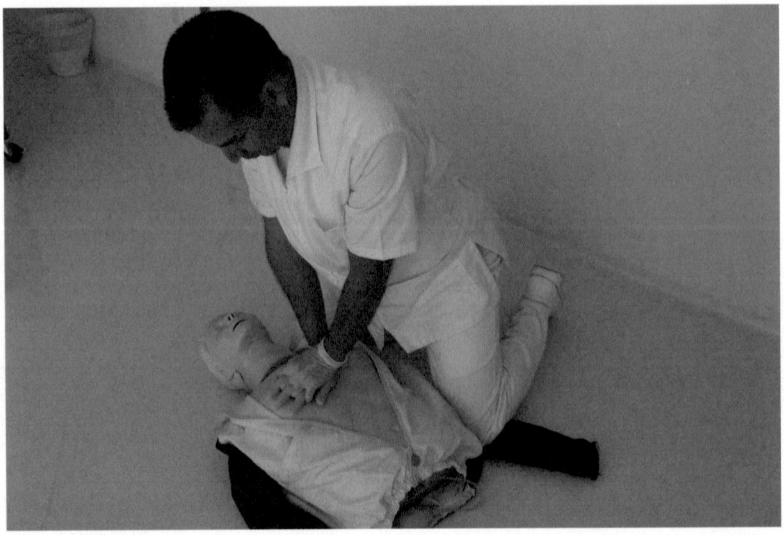

Figure 4-13. The glance should fall naturally on the contrary side of the victim, to help in maintaining an adequate position during the thoracic compressions.

Prior to evaluating the pulse and the breathing, five cycles of 30 thoracic compressions will be completed for every two ventilations. The steps for CPR can be summed up in an algorithm to integrate the knowledge and direct the sequence of action (Figure 4-14).

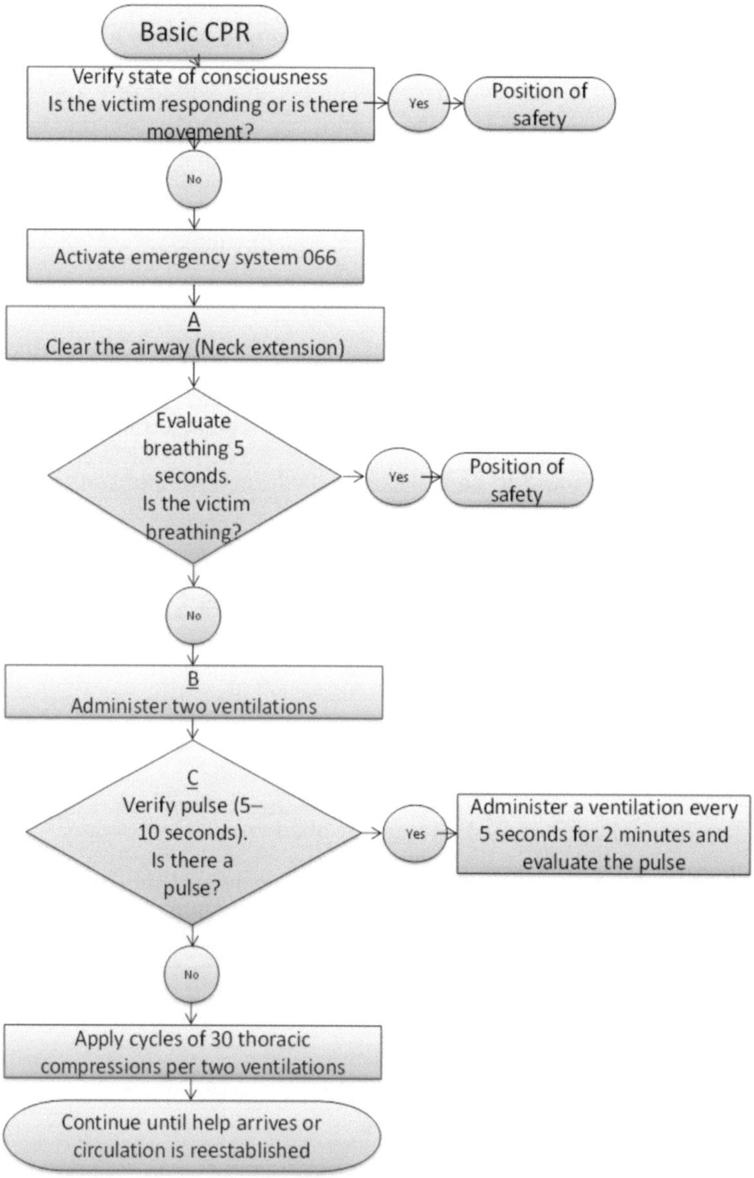

Figure 4-14. Algorithm for Basic cardiopulmonary resuscitation (CPR-B).

Conditions for initiating or delaying cardiopulmonary resuscitation

It should be clarified that it is the responsibility of the health personnel to provide resuscitation maneuvers to each person who presents Respiratory arrest (RA); it is noteworthy that there are situations in which no intervention can be performed. Mention is made briefly of some of these as follows:

- That death is evident, as in the case of some traumatic mutilation that definitively is not compatible with life; a massive hemorrhage or, for example, signs of lividity or rigor mortis.
- When our lives as assistants are in danger; remember that within pre-hospitalary care, we must add the primary evaluation that, in addition to identifying data that can be useful to assess our patient, has as its purpose the detection of potential risks for our own integrity. A dead or injured assistant has no value.
- When someone with the faculties to do so certifies the death.
- When the cardiac and respiratory function reestablishes spontaneously after applying the maneuvers.
- When the responsibility of care is transferred to other assistants, whether equally or more extensively trained, at the site of the accident or in a specialized unit.
- When the assistants are found to be truly exhausted, incapable of continuing to provide resuscitation maneuvers.

At present and based on revisions carried out on basic life-support protocols, additional criteria have been added in relation to the ceasing of efforts during CPR. It is necessary for the following to present together in order to justify stopping the maneuvers.

- If the CRA did not occur in the presence of some assistant.
- If the victim's cardiac and respiratory function was not reestablished after three cycles of CPR.
- Finally, if the patient did not have discharges applied with a Defibrillator.

If these three criteria are complied with, it would be considered timely to stop the maneuvers.

Chapter 5

2010 Update of the American Heart Association (AHA) Guidelines

In the latest edition of the AHA Guidelines, substantial changes were made to the protocols, in the execution of maneuvers as well as in the requirements of the maneuvers.

One aspect that is proposed is quality CPR, with attention to the following aspects:

- Frequency in compressions of at least 100 per minute. In the former guidelines, it was proposed for this to be approximately 100 compressions per minute. It was identified that the compressions that are applied are determining for survival. Formerly, the number of compressions proposed, counting the interruptions that can present during the sequence, was not always covered.
- Depth of compressions should be 5 cm in adults and one third of the thoracic diameter in children and infants. Adequate perfusion is achieved through thoracic compression; in many cases, the compression was not sufficiently strong because it ranged in depth from 4–5 cm and did not always comply with the requirements.
- Decrease interruptions as much as possible during the thoracic compressions.
- Permit complete thoracic expansion after each compression.
- Avoid excessive ventilation.
- A complication that can present is gastric distension, vomiting (emesis), and aspiration of the contents.

The A-B-C sequence is exchanged for C-A-B

Customarily, the sequence was known as A-B-C and was very useful, but it was observed that in the majority of cases, a victim of Cardiorespiratory arrest (CRA) was found by witnesses not to have had thoracic compressions applied, for diverse reasons, such as fear of the legal repercussions that could exist, total ignorance concerning what to do, because for persons not familiarized with the health area it can be very complex to execute the steps comprising traditional CPR.

It is not easy to assess breathing, the pulse, or simply to permeabilize the airways; due to these doubts, time is lost for implementing thoracic compressions. With the exchange in A-B-C sequence for C-B-A, time is not lost in applying the compressions, which are of vital importance and the delay in ventilation is not too great.

LEGO resuscitator

The concept of the Locally Enabled, Globally Optimized (LEGO) resuscitator is introduced, including a simplified algorithm, whose purpose is to simplify CPR, placing emphasis on the thoracic compressions. The sequence includes the following:

- Assess the victim's state of consciousness or the victim's response.
- Assess briefly whether breathing is present. If there is gasping for breath or blockage, the **S**eeing, **H**earing, and **F**eeling (**SHF**) technique is eliminated.
- The Emergency medical service (EMS) is activated.
- If available, use an Automatic external defibrillator (AED). If not, request one.
- Initiate thoracic compressions at a rhythm of at least 100 per minute, with a depth of 5 cm.
- If the resuscitator possesses the ability and training, the airway should be opened and two ventilations should be applied, with a 1-second duration, after every 30 compressions.
- If the resuscitator does not know how to or cannot perform this, continue applying thoracic compressions until the AED or the emergency personnel arrives.

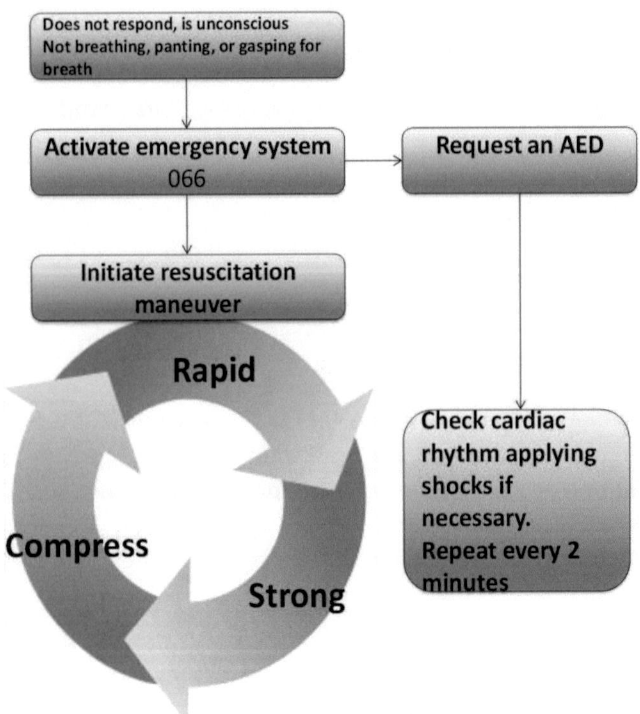

Figure 5-1. Algorithm for LEGO resuscitators.

Although the LEGO algorithm for resuscitators (Figure 5-1) is simpler, the AHA states that persons with training in CPR should learn the complete method, taking into consideration that the thoracic compressions and the rescue ventilations continue to comprise the preferred techniques for CPR.

The AHA also cites that the teaching of compressions-only CPR is an alternative solely for persons without contact with the health area, or for those who are not willing to learn the complete technique.

Chapter 6

Clearing the Airways of a Foreign Body

Airway obstruction is commonly known as choking. This emergency situation is generated when some foreign object occludes these, impeding the passage of air in both directions.

The obstruction can be partial or total. Partial obstruction allows the passage of a small amount of air; thus, the victim can generate audible noises, faltering speech, or cough, in which case the victim should only be supported so as to cough up the object him/herself and restart his/her breathing correctly. In these cases, it is useful to be supported by the assisted-coughing technique, so that together with maximum inspiration and abdominal pressure, the airway may be cleared. In the case of total obstruction, the victim is unable to emit any sound, including the voice, due to that these are generated by the free passage of air through the throat.

Heimlich maneuver

The method recommended for counteracting asphyxia is the Heimlich maneuver, named for Dr. Henry Heimlich, who implemented it for the first time in 1974.

- Initial management of the situation lies in identifying the obstruction; we generally identify in the victim the "universal choking sign" (Figure 6-1), which consists of raising the hands to the throat in a gesture of anguish.
- After this, an approximation to the victim is made, with the responder in front in the victim's visual field; we take the victim by the shoulders and ask him/her: Can you speak? Can you cough? If the victim does not respond or does not emit any sound, we find ourselves in effect in the face of total airways obstruction (Figure 6-2).
- We should place ourselves behind the victim and embrace him/her with both arms, placing our little finger in the umbilicus and our thumb on the xiphoid appendix (Figure 6-3) to determine the midpoint between these two sites, then placing the same hand at the midpoint in a fist (Figure 6-4).
- Next, place the other hand over the first and begin compressions on the abdomen in ascending fashion, as if tracing the letter "J" (Figure 6-5).
- Continue the compressions until the victim expels the foreign body or loses consciousness.

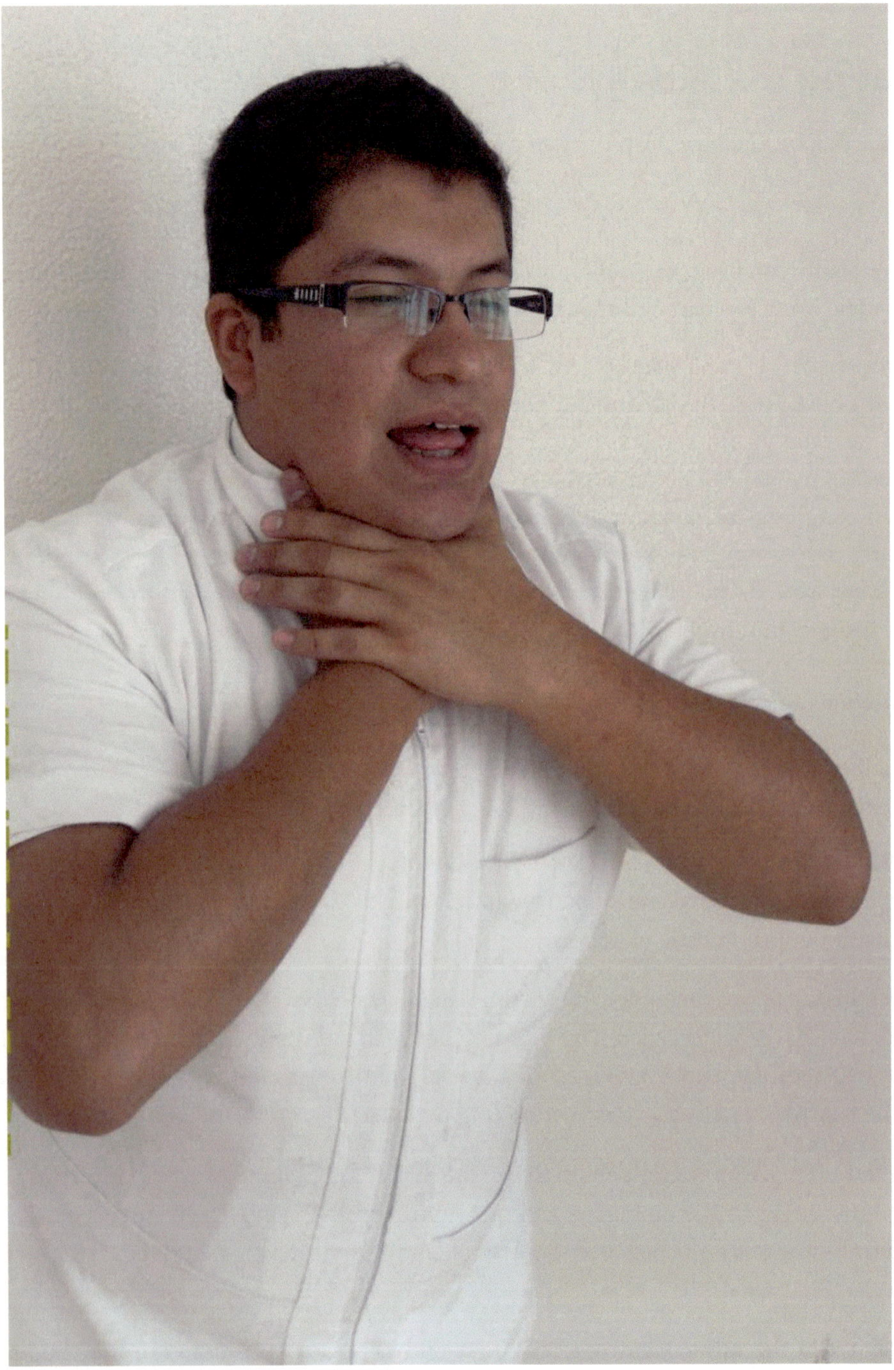

Figure 6-1. The image depicts a person who presents airway obstruction, who by reflex, raises the hands to the neck, which is known as the "universal choking sign".

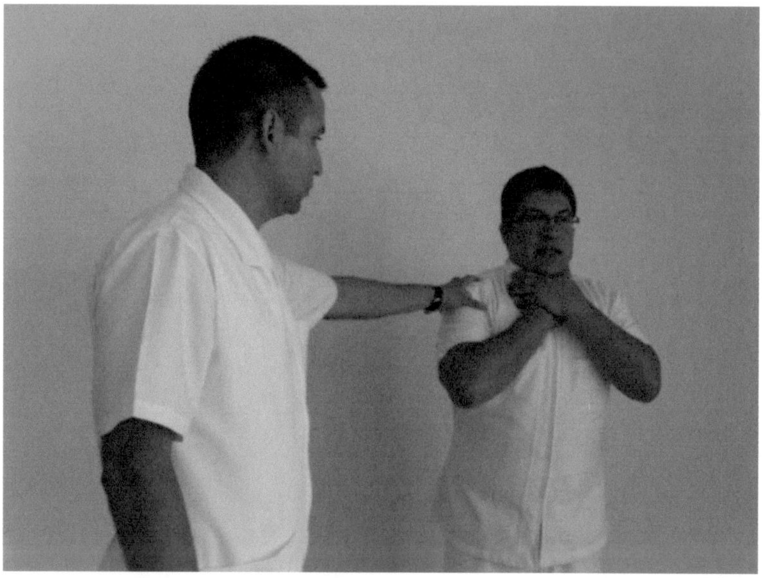

Figure 6-2. The correct way to approach the victim. In the face of this type of situation, it is important to be assertive on identifying what is happening; if we approach the person who is choking from behind, it can increase their anxiety and avoid their cooperating with us.

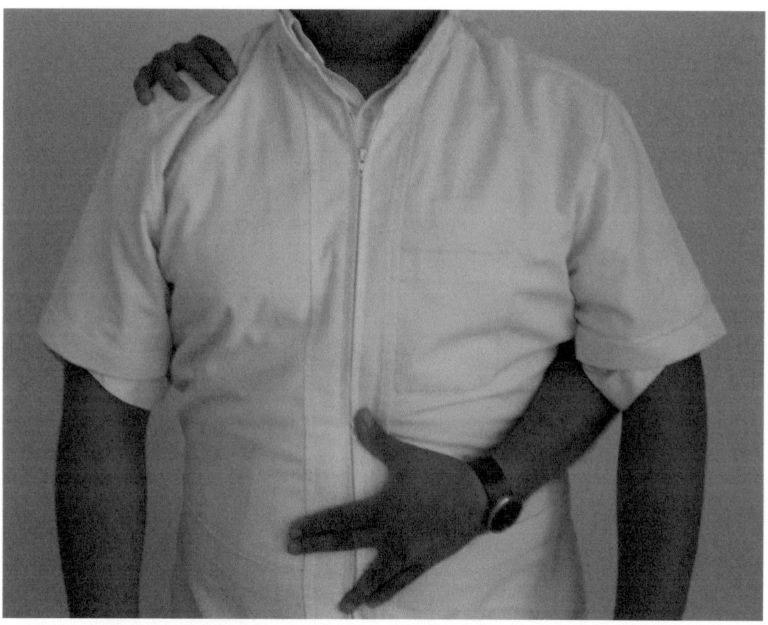

Figure 6-3. Place the thumb on the xiphoid appendix. In the case of not localizing the umbilicus (that is utilized as the anatomical reference), the little fingers is situated on the waist or where the where the belt buckle would be.

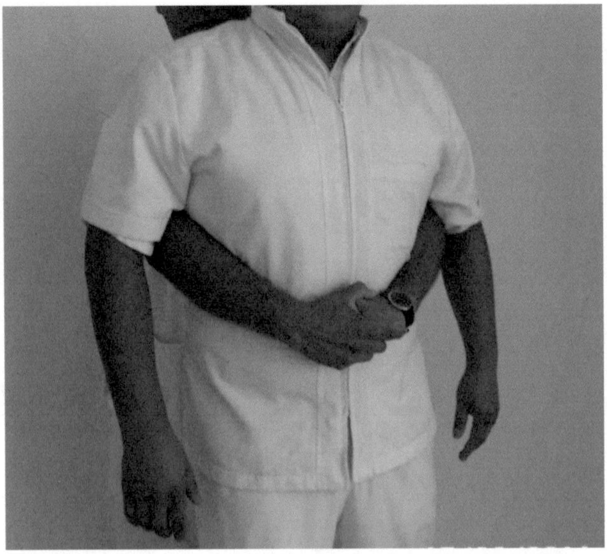

Figure 6-4. One hand should be placed over the other, the first should be in a fist and the second should be extended to exert pressure.

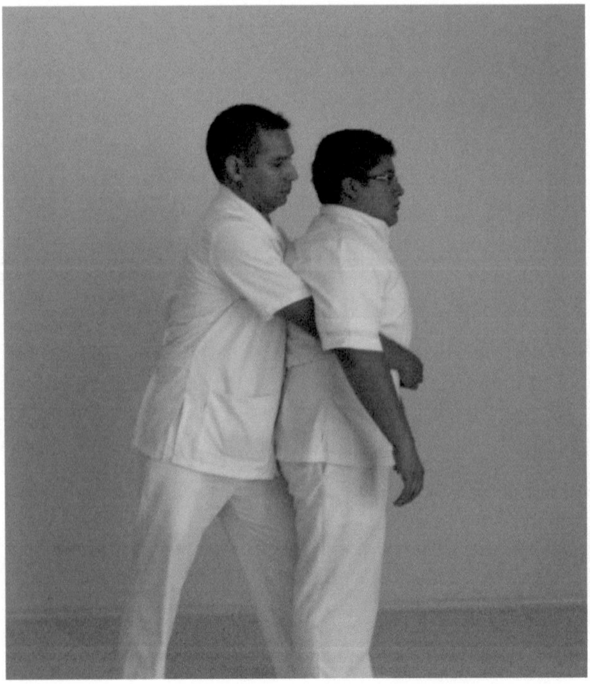

Figure 6-5. The correct position to carry out the compressions. The procedure permits the foreign object to be expelled by air, by the contents of the stomach, or by the compression on the diaphragm.

Unconscious victim

In general, the majority of persons lose consciousness after 90 seconds of being unable to breathe. If the victim is found in this situation, it is deduced that the loss of consciousness is caused by asphyxia. Therefore, treatment should be continued in the following manner:

- The airway should be opened to attempt to localize the foreign body and, if possible, to remove it (Figure 6-6). If the foreign body cannot be seen, the fingers should not be introduced in an attempt to localize it; this could be harmful because the foreign object can be pushed and lodged to an even greater degree.
- Next, Cardiopulmonary resuscitation (CPR) maneuvers should be initiated as described previously.
- During resuscitation maneuvers, each time the airway is opened to ventilate, the resuscitator should verify whether the foreign body can be observed; if so, try to extract it. If this is not possible, continue.

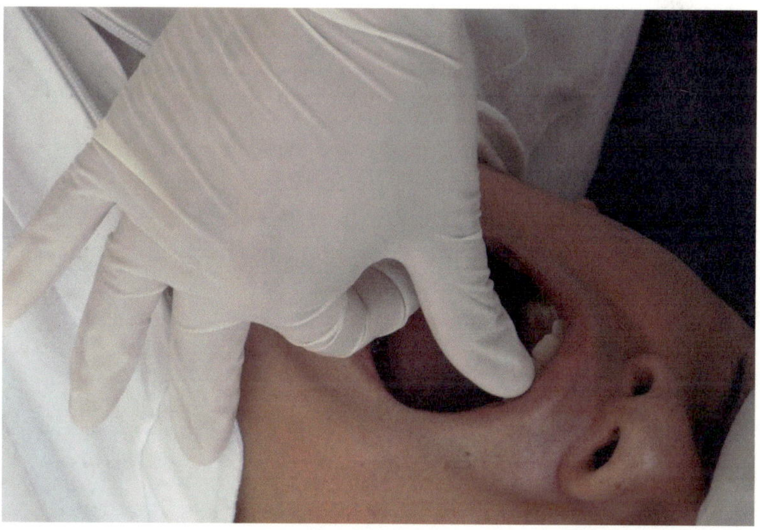

Figure 6-6. The correct way of carrying out the "crossed- fingers" technique, in which the point of the thumbs and index fingers should be placed along the front teeth, without introducing them completely into the mouth, and then making a movement as if snapping the fingers, to observe the interior of the mouth without the risk of being bitten.

Reestablishment of the airway

If as a consequence of the maneuvers unblocking the airway is achieved, this can be identified in the following ways:

- It is observed that the victim expels the object during the compressions.
- Free passage of air is perceived and thoracic expansion is observed on insufflating.

In this case, we should:

- Give two deep insufflations.
- Verify the pulse for 5 seconds, no more than 10.
- Depending on the result, incorporate the mouth-to-mouth resuscitation technique, thoracic compressions, or simply the position of safety.

The maneuver for clearing the airways is performed following the steps by means of an algorithm (Figure 6-7).

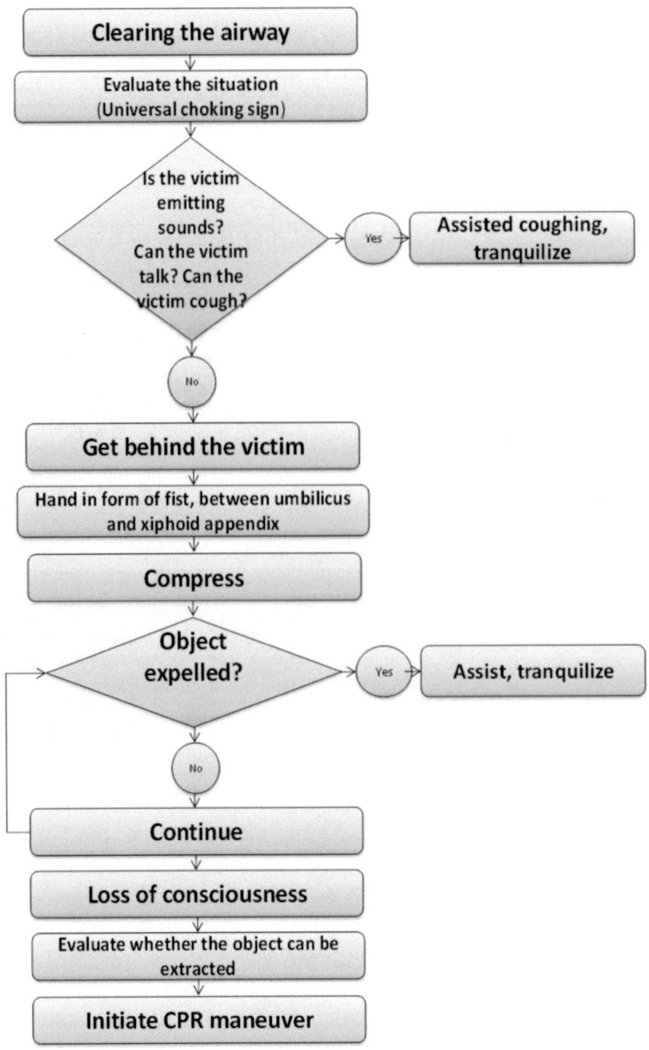

Figure 6-7. Algorithm to unblock the airway due to a foreign body.

Special considerations

There are some situations that can create confusion in the assistant and that generate modifications in the technique:

- Pregnant women and very obese persons. In these cases, the abdominal compressions are exchanged for thoracic compressions, placing the arms in the same way around the victim underneath the armpits, in the same site as for CPR.
- When a person him/herself is the victim and is alone, one should find the way to effect the compressions on oneself, supporting oneself on a blunt object, for example, a table or a chair.

Clearing the airways and liquids

In the previous chapters, we described in detail the simple and basic notions of acting at the first moment of Cardiorespiratory arrest (CRA) associated with the aspiration of solid foreign objects present in the airways. However, it is necessary to ask oneself, *What if the airways obstruction is due to liquids?*

The airway and the digestive tract have common cavities; thus, during eating, precisely at the moment that the food bolus or the swallowing of some liquid is to be ingested, the person may take a breath and part of the ingested bolus or liquid go toward the airway, causing a protector reflex, occluding the opening of the glottis, in turn blocking breathing. This occlusion reflex of the glottis is produced by the contraction of the abductors and inhibition of the adductors, a strong laryngeal stimulation that can even lead to a laryngospasm or prolonged bronchoconstriction. In these cases, one must act rapidly and precisely, because if not, Cardiopulmonary arrest (CPA) will be produced.

On first intent, the cough reflex should be obtained, given that it is a protector reflex in which the larynx and glottis are involved. Coughing is a highly important mechanism, because it carries out to a great degree the cleaning of the tracheobronchial tree, promoting lung expansion. Together with the capacity to generate forced coughing (gagging), it is a coadjutant in the effort of airway permeability, at the same time that the liquid found in the airway and/or that has generated the glottis' closing reflex is expelled. On the other hand, if the closure of the glottis continues, if the liquid is not expelled, and coughing as a tracheobronchial tree cleaning mechanism is not achieved, the victim will inevitably fall into apnea, thus into Cardiopulmonary arrest (CPA). If this occurs, the CPR-B protocol should be initiated.

Chapter 7

Clearing the Airways in Children

Upper airway obstruction constitutes one of the most frequent emergencies in children that require immediate attention because it is a severe problem that causes serious breathing complications and that at the same time evolves very rapidly into hypoxia, thus producing death, or failing that, quite severe and definitive neurological sequelae.

The risk of airways obstruction in infants and children is more frequent than in the adult, due to the characteristics of the anatomical structures in their airway, given that its diameter is very small, above all below the glottis, with the epiglottis larger and the trachea, smaller. Therefore, there is more danger in children. When obstruction is present, edema is also generally present, which reduces the lumen by >30%. This reduction renders the child unable to tolerate this problem.

Among the multiple causes that can bring about an airways obstruction, we find the following:

1. Injuries due to burns in the respiratory airway.
2. Some diseases such as tracheititis.
3. The presence of some foreign body.
4. Aspiration of a liquid.
5. Airway trauma.
6. Inhalation of toxic gases.

Therefore, assistance, help, or care must be immediate, that is, with initial management. In addition, it must be correct because if it is delayed or if errors are committed, Cardiorespiratory arrest (CRA) is accelerated. Due to all of these elements, there should be awareness of the importance of this immediate and correct initial management for non-expert individuals as well as for those with experience in the management of cases. What is important is to act with the purpose of clearing the airway and for this, there must be an extra- and intra-hospitalary management plan in place,

The purpose of the plan consists of carrying out maneuvers so that the child is disturbed to the least extent possible. The obstruction that presents most frequently is the aspiration of a foreign body that causes partial (less serious) or total (severe) obstruction. The latter causes more deaths in children, above all in those aged <3 years. The products aspirated, such as small toys or small pieces of larger toys that are plastic or metal, liquids, foods, dry fruit seeds such as nuts, peanuts, etc., can become lodged in the pharynx, trachea, and bronchi, this latter place the most frequent for these to be become lodged. The child suddenly presents choking data that are recognized by episodes of acute coughing, nausea that can lead to vomiting, and difficulty in breathing, which causes a bluish coloration of the skin (cyanosis), triggering intense and persistent coughing. The signs and symptoms of upper airway obstruction will vary depending on the degree of obstruction. If the obstruction is incomplete, there will be coughing and stridency on inspiration. If, on the other hand, the obstruction is complete, it will produce severe asphyxia and Cardiopulmonary arrest (PCR) if the airway is not unblocked rapidly.

The assistant must be seated or kneeling in order to hold the infant down safely on the his/her forearm, holding the infant's head and placing the thumb of one hand at an angle to the jaw and one or two fingers of the same hand at the angle contrary to the jaw. The soft tissues under the infant's jaw should not be compressed, because this could exacerbate the airway obstruction. Apply up to five sharp blows to the infant's back with the heel of the other hand on the infant's back midway between the shoulder blades (Figure 7-1).

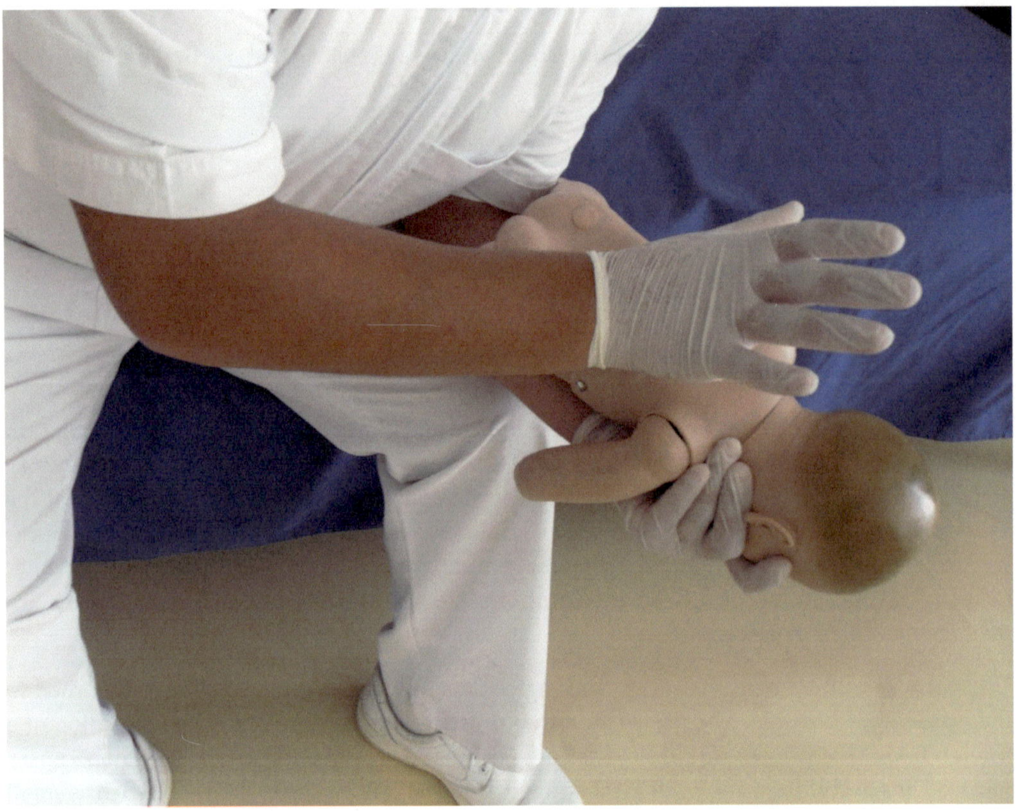

Figure 7-1. Clearing the airway. The image shows us the correct way to perform cleaning of the airway.

If the blows to the infant's back cannot expel the object and the infant remains conscious, the assistant will proceed to carry out thoracic compressions. The Heimlich maneuver should not be employed at any time in children < 1 year of age.

When this type of maneuver does not correct the obstruction problems, the child should be transferred to a health institution where other methods to assess the problem will be utilized by professionals who are experts in this type of situation. A careful exploratory examination will be conducted and some imaging studies, ranging from the most simple to the most complex. If the obstruction is partial, radiographs will be carried out with x-rays taken lateral to the neck and thorax, and on some occasions, removal of the foreign body will be required under the effects of anesthesia by means of bronchoscopy in the operating room. If complete obstruction is present, more complex unblocking maneuvers must be performed.

Chapter 8

Basic Cardiopulmonary Resuscitation in Infants

This is the procedure that involves a set of maneuvers to correct Cardiorespiratory arrest (CRA). The situations that lead to CRA in children under 1 year of age are as follows: choking; asphyxia; craniocephalic trauma; serious injuries; hemorrhages; electrical discharges, and intoxication. The symptoms are as follows: loss of consciousness; absence of breathing, and absence of a pulse.

Airway management

Management of the airways acquires notable relevance in the treatment of trauma victims. The inability that the victims undergo in maintaining correct oxygenation and ventilation causes secondary brain injuries, with a greater risk than primary injuries, thus the importance of guaranteeing correct permeability of the airways and maintaining oxygenation of the victim during the time that ventilatory support is provided if necessary. It is essential to diminish the probabilities of brain damage. Correct airways management, for an optimal contribution of oxygen to the body as well as to the brain, constitutes an essential component in pre-hospitalary care.

The most common causes that can affect the capacity of the respiratory apparatus

1. Hypoventilation or loss of ventilation. This occurs due to alteration of the state of consciousness, above all to traumatic brain injury. Obstruction of the airways due to a foreign object or aspiration of a liquid.

2. Hypoventilation due to reduction of lung expansion.

3. Hypoxia that can be caused by diminution of hemorrhage-associated blood flow.

4. Another reason that can lead to hypoxia is that the alveoli are filled with liquid or another residue.

Alteration in the state of consciousness

In an unconscious victim, the primary cause of airway obstruction is due to the tongue, which has lost its muscle tone and tends to retract, obstructing the airways and impeding the passage of oxygen to the trachea and lungs.

Control of the Airways (A)

Ensuring a permeable airway is the first priority in the treatment and resuscitation of victims, and nothing is more important than a correct evaluation in pre-hospitalary care.

Manual unblocking of the airways

Prior to performing any technique on the victim, the oropharyngeal cavity should be evaluated visually and rapidly; the purpose of this is to find any foreign body in the mouth. This can be extracted manually with the greatest safety and hygiene possible.

Manual maneuvers

In unconscious pediatric victims, the techniques that should be used are the following:

1. Modified triple maneuver (Figure 8-1).

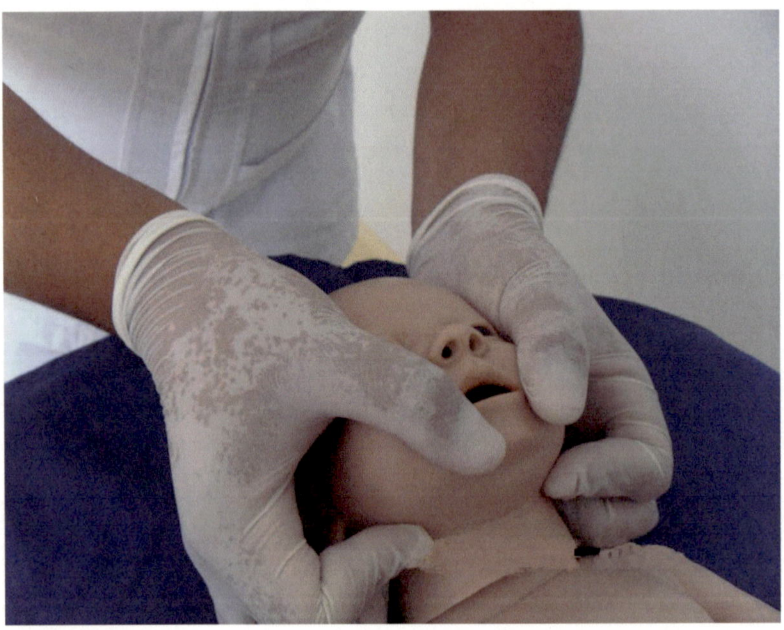

Figure 8-1. Modified triple maneuver in which the index and middle fingers are placed under the mandible and the thumb beyond the level of the lower incisors, so as to afterward raise the chin with displacement of the tongue toward a more backward position and unblock the airway.

This consists of positioning the jaw in a slight extension at an angle of approximately 30º with respect to the head, placing the index and middle fingers in the forward region of the chin and the thumbs on the lips at the level of the lower incisors. In this position, the assistant will proceed to make an extension (traction toward the apex), with which the placement of the base of the tongue in a vertical or anterior position is achieved, thus unblocking the airway.

2. Jaw displacement.

Mouth-to-mouth breathing (B)

In pediatric victims, unlike adult victims, mouth-to-mouth resuscitation is performed by covering the mouth and the nose in their totality. In these insufflations, only the air contained in the mouth of the assistant will be applied (Figure 8-2).

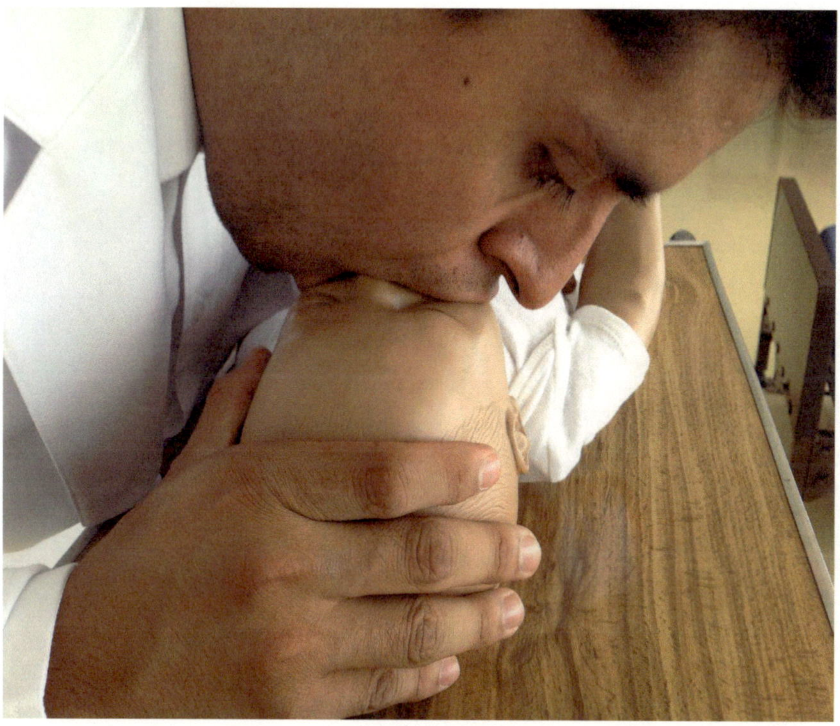

Figure 8-2. Correct way to perform mouth-to-mouth resuscitation in infants.

Circulation – Cardiac massage (C)

In victims younger than 1 year of age, there is a great difference in the sequence of the application of compressions (Figure 8-3). Compressions in victims under 1 year of age will be performed with the force of two fingers above the xiphoid appendix and compressing to a depth of approximately 4 centimeters (Figure 8-4).

It is noteworthy that if one does not have adequate training in CPR, the maneuvers should not be suspended until specialized personnel arrive on the scene.

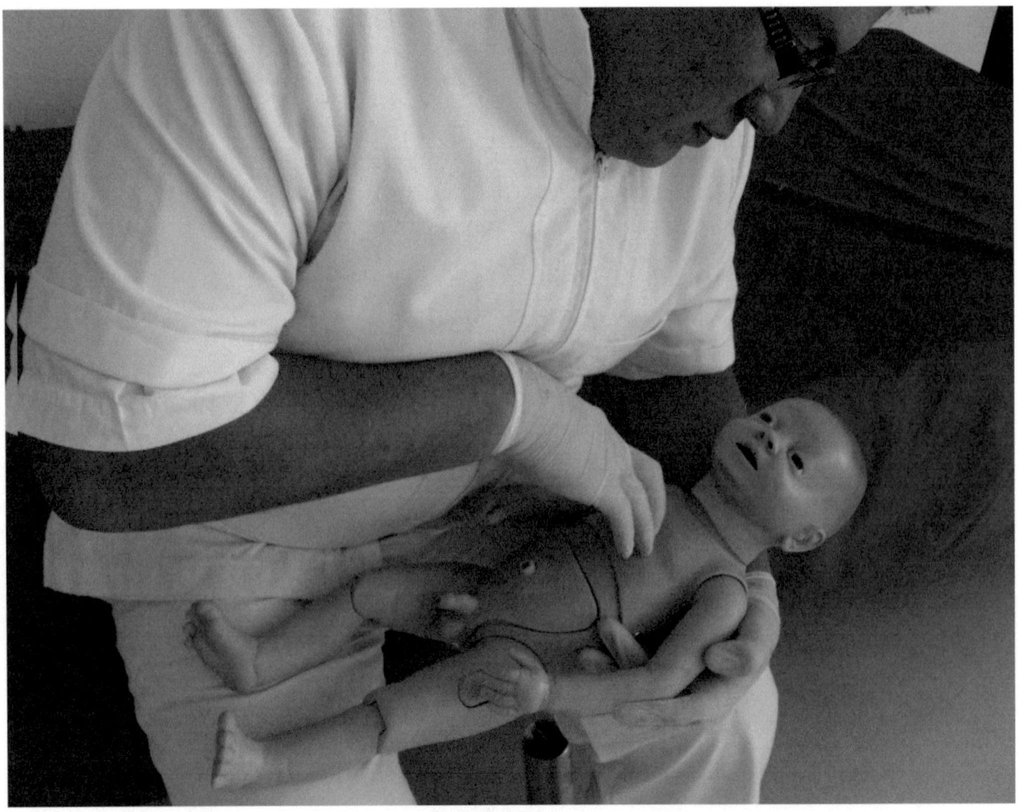

Figure 8-3. Way to place the infant to perform compressions and to localize the correct compression point

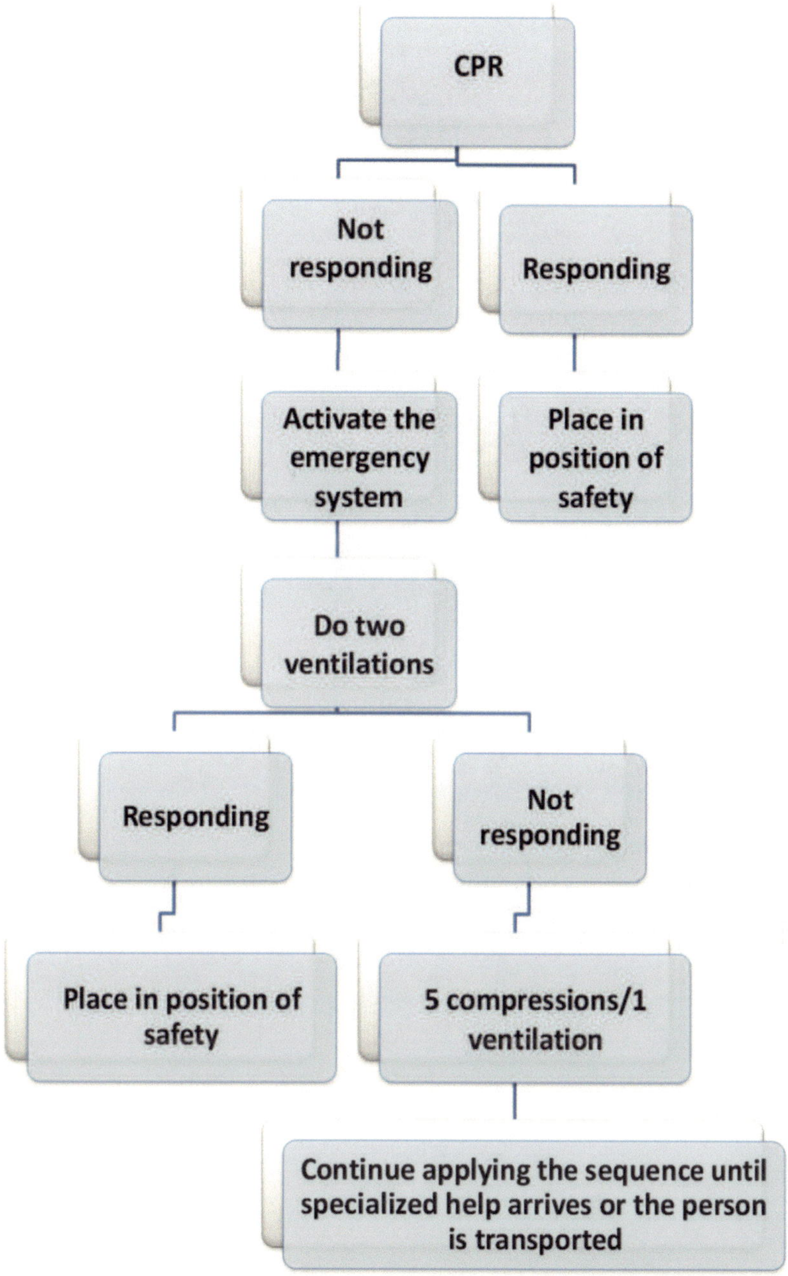

Figure 8-4. Resuscitation algorithm

Position of safety. This position allows us better management of the victim, thus avoiding greater injury to him/her (Figure 8-5). As is well known, pre-hospitalary care has as its final purpose, above all, not to cause more harm to the victim.

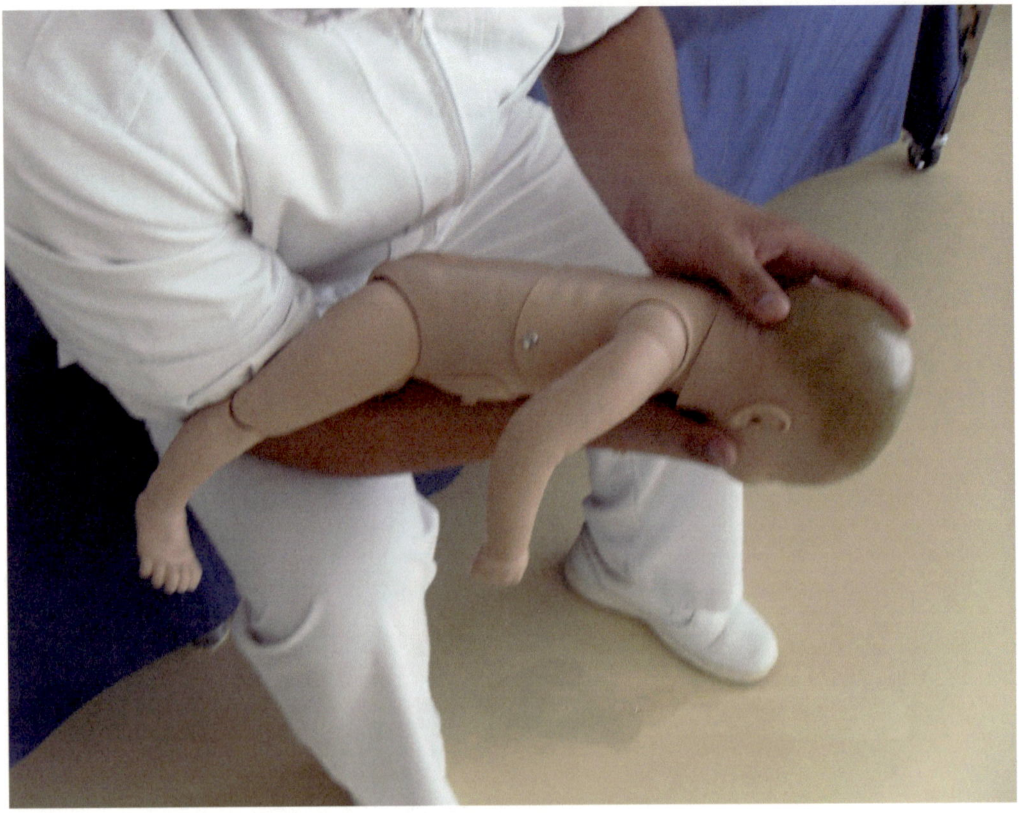

Figure 8-5. Correct way to place the infant in a position of safety.

Chapter 9

Cardiopulmonary Resuscitation in Pregnant Women

Gestation is a physiological process; therefore, the birth of a healthy child is an event that is traditionally celebrated in all societies worldwide. This event signifies the successful culmination of the reproductive process with positive results in terms of the survival and well-being of the trinome.

However, in many cases, the reproductive process become a high-risk event that can result in morbility and mortality in the mother and the product. During pregnancy, many physiological changes take place that cause some symptoms and discomfort. The greater part of these discomforts do not require the application of any therapeutic measure; however, the pregnant women requires an explanation to calm her because in the majority of women, the seriousness of some symptom in particular cannot be assessed, which can complicate the pregnancy, such as CRA, placing the binome at risk.

During pregnancy, it is estimated that CRA presents in one of every 30,000 pregnancies; survival of the pregnancy is 7%. It is considered that the key to resuscitating the product is resuscitating the mother. The key intervention in the prevention of CRA in the pregnant woman in a critical state is positioning her on her left lateral decubitus (modified 30º), supplementary oxygen, valvular access, evaluating the pressure numbers, and considering the possible reversible causes. Here we make known the main causes for which pregnant women fall into Cardiorespiratory arrest: thromboembolism; sepsis, pregnancy-induced hypertension; amniotic liquid embolism; placenta abruptio; placenta previa; uterine atony; Disseminated intravascular coagulation (DIC); hypermagnesemia; drug errors or allergies; trauma; anesthesia complications; baseline cardiopathies, and congenital or acquired causes.

Among the physiological changes in advanced pregnancy that affect CPR are the respiratory changes, among these the following: increase in ventilation; increase in the demand for oxygen, and reduction in thoracic distensibility, and reduction in the functional reserve capacity. Among the cardiovascular changes, we find the following: incomplete gastroesophageal sphincter; increase in intra-gastric pressure, and an increase in the risk of regurgitation.

Cardiovascular PCR in pregnant patients corresponds to an infrequent event with which obstetricians, physicians, and nursing professionals may be faced at some moment in their career, given that the results depend on the underlying cause of the arrest and the rapidity of the resuscitation efforts, which requires a basic knowledge of the principles of resuscitation as well as of the peculiarities of the latter, within the context of the CRA of a pregnant woman. During the resuscitation attempt of a pregnant woman, two patients are involved: the mother and the product, with maternal survival the best hope for fetal survival.

Recommendations for carrying out CPR during pregnancy consider that the incidence of arrest during gestation is one case per every 30,000 pregnancies. Despite that the incidence of Cardiorespiratory arrest in the pregnant woman is infrequent, the possibility of resuscitating her is relatively low; thus, it is important that the entire multidisciplinary team know what to do to offer the binome quality care and safety, taking into consideration the existence of respiratory, circulatory, gastrointestinal, and metabolic changes that have direct implications on the CPR, which will lead to the possibility of performing a cesarean taking into account the product's gestational age in weeks.

In pregnancy, the causes that produce CRA are different in relation to any other victim. Independently of the causes, poor ventilation technique produces cerebral hypofusion that leads to tissue anoxia; thus, action should be taken rapidly and in an adequate manner. Cardiopulmonary or cardiorespiratory arrest is the most serious event that can present in an obstetric emergency; it requires immediate and correct attention to avoid the death of the victim or of the victim's remaining with irreversible neurological sequelae.

Successful resuscitation of a pregnant woman and survival of the fetus require timely and excellent CPR, in addition to some modifications in technique. At week 20 of gestation, the gravid uterus can compress the inferior vena cava and the aorta, obstructing venous return and arterial flow. Resuscitators can relieve this compression by placing the patient in left lateral decubitus position, or by pushing the uterus sideways.

The defibrillation and the drug dose employed for resuscitation of the pregnant woman are the same as those utilized for adults with CRA. It is noteworthy that cardioversion appears to be safe for the fetus. Resuscitators should consider the need for a peri-mortem cesarean as soon as the pregnant woman develops cardiaç arrest, and should be prepared to proceed with hysterectomy if resuscitation is unsuccessful in the course of a few minutes.

Primary A-B-C-D in pregnant women

A. **Airway**. In order to ensure a permeable airway, an advanced add-on device should be inserted to reduce the risk of regurgitation and/or aspiration. Airway edema and spasm can reduce the diameter of the trachea; the resuscitator should be ready to use an endotracheal tube, monitoring bleeding after the insertion of any tube within the oropharynx or nasopharynx, which should be placed by an expert. Oxygenation is a priority because hypoxia can present rapidly; intubation is of rapid sequence with cricoidal pressure, and agents should be selected for anesthesia or deep sedation to minimize hypotension.

B. **Ventilation**. Without modifications in confirmation of placement of the tube. Taking into account that the gravid uterus raises the diaphragm and that pulmonary function is found to be compromised, causing that the patient can develop hypoxia.

C. **External thoracic compressions**. The patient should be placed in the left lateral position at an angle of between 15 and 30º, with uterine displacement, afterward initiating the thoracic compressions at a rate of 30 compressions per 2 ventilations per 5 cycles. A thin metal support device should be placed under the right side (allowing the patient to recline in her left side) or for the resuscitator to kneel near the patient's left side, in such a way that traction is made and the gravid uterus decompresses the inferior vena cava.

D. **Defibrillation**. Without modification neither in dose nor in the placement site of the paddles. The discharge does not affect the product, because the defibrillation discharges do not transfer significant currents to the fetus. All fetal monitoring devices should be removed prior to the discharge.

CRA in pregnant women requires special considerations due to the fact that two lives are involved.

In the normal pregnancy, cardiac expenditure and blood volume increase >50%.In addition, there is an increase in cardiac frequency, respiratory frequency, and in oxygen pulmonary residual functional capacity, as well as in peripheral and pulmonary vascular resistance. Taken together, all of these alterations render the pregnant woman more fragile to cardiovascular and respiratory changes.

Another important critical factor that exerts an impact on the effectiveness of CPR and on hemodynamic support in pregnant patients is the aortocaval compression produced by the gravid uterus during the second half of the pregnancy. In advanced pregnancy, the vena cava can be completely obstructed. In the majority of women in the supine position, venous return is forced through the lumbar azygos veins and the paraspinal veins. Around 10% of pregnant women manifest the supine hypotension syndrome, in which syncope, hypotension, and brachycardia present, due to aortocaval compression. Systolic volume and cardiac expenditure increase between 25 and 30% when pregnant patients in the third trimester go from a supine to a lateral position.

The respiratory changes of pregnancy include the increase of thoracic expansions per minute, caused by the effects of progesterone on the respiratory center, the increase of oxygen consumption, and the restrictive ventilatory defect caused by cranial displacement of the diaphragm. Arterial gasometry during the at-term pregnancy tends to reflect a state of respiratory compensated alkalosis. The mechanical effects of gravid uterus and the hypertrophic breasts give rise to a reduction in the functional reserve capacity and a reduction in thoracic wall distensibility. Reduction in functional reserve capacity, and increased oxygen consumption can precipitate oxygen desaturation if hypoventilation is produced.

It is essential to know the respiratory changes of pregnancy during the treatment of CRA. These changes require the rapid reestablishment of oxygenation and of ventilation. Increased oxygen consumption leads to greater frequencies of arterial oxygen desaturation in the peri-partum woman found with apnea.

Prior to week 24 of gestation, in CRA, the main objective of resuscitators will be to save the life of the mother, because the fetus will have many more possibilities of survival, because from this date the fetus is estimated to be more viable. Beyond week 24 of gestation, and together with that of the mother, the life of the fetus should be considered as potentially viable. Apply management algorithms of Cardiac life support (CLS) and Assisted ventilatory support (AVS), Advanced cardiac life support (ACLS), to victims of Cardiac arrest (CA) according to four key modifications as follows:

1. Airways management.
2. Uterine displacement.
3. Deeper external thoracic compressions.
4. Peri-partum delivery care within the first 5 minutes post-partum.

Maternal benefits after rapid CPR

1. Aortocaval compression disappears.
2. Increase of venous return.
3. Increase in the effectiveness of external thoracic compressions.
4. Increase of between 25 and 33% in post-load after external thoracic compressions.

Chapter 10

Ethical and Legal Aspects in Basic Cardiopulmonary Resuscitation

Ethics is a discipline that studies human behavior from a normative action mode; this, it is important to remember that humans have rights and the first of these contemplates the right to a dignified life and a dignified death.

The intent of basic cardiopulmonary resuscitation is to initiate the rescue of the victim by any person with learning and training; thus, the ethics applied to this act is considered positive judgment due to the intent to recover the life that is being lost and the person's act is considered to entertain a good purpose because it clearly favors life.

Basic CPR is a series of procedures and techniques based on guidelines and protocols, but that are conducted in an unfavorable environment, and in some situations the decisions that must be made possess a great moral component. These should be based on the principles of autonomy, beneficence, and distributive justice as designated in the ethical code for the nursing professional.

It is very important to determine when these CPR techniques are to be applied and the time to continue to follow these. In this situation, it is fundamental to remember the two ethical principles of life, precisely the right to a dignified life and a dignified death, with the acceptance of an irreversible process that leads to death.

When to initiate CPR?

a. When there are possibilities of recovering the victim's vital functions.

b. When there is no vital danger for the resuscitator.

c. When we do not know or when there exists a reasonable doubt concerning the characteristics of the patient and/or of the time and circumstances of the cardiorespiratory arrest.

When should CPR not be initiated?

a. When the time period of the cardiorespiratory arrest is not known, but there are evident signs of biological death.

b. When the cardiorespiratory arrest is the natural evolution of a disease without the possibilities of treatment.

When should CPR be finalized?

1. When the time that has transpired is >10 minutes from the arrest and the initiation of CPR with a positive response from the victim.
2. When the victim presents signs of biological death. 1
3. When 10 minutes have transpired from the beginning of CPR without any assistance from or any positive response by the victim.
4. When the resuscitation has been effective, with the recovery of spontaneous circulation and respiration.
5. When there is serious risk for other victims or the resuscitator.
6. When the responsibility is transferred to a more experienced person.

It is important to remember that a code of professional ethics is a document that clearly establishes the moral principles, duties, and obligations that guide professional performance. This code demands excellence in standards of practice and maintains a strict relationship with the law of the professional exercise that determines the minimally accepted norms to avoid discrepancies.

It is noteworthy that the observance of ethical norms in health professionals is a personal responsibility, one of conscience and of the will to be at peace with oneself. A code of ethics makes explicit the prime purposes, the values, and the obligations that inspire respect for life, for health, and for death as marked by the ethical code for nurses of both genders in Mexico.

In Mexico, this initiates with the teaching of Cerebral cardiopulmonary resuscitation (CCPR) in an obligatory manner with the members of the health team, considering that the community in general possesses little or null knowledge of the maneuvers that should be performed in an accident, and it is very important to initiate training the population in the maneuvers that should be carried out in an accident. It is fundamental for all health professionals and student to have knowledge, training, and updating of basic CPR.

Legal aspects in cardiopulmonary resuscitation

The application of CPR maneuvers can generate medical-legal consequences. If the patient survives, he/she has the right to the information. But if the patient dies, the information should be integrated into the diagnosis of death by means of the autopsy, which will determine the causes.

It is easy to fall into what is known as the "technological imperative", that is, to do everything that can be done. In this situation, it is possible to act due to fear of legal negligence or a legal claim at a later date, because health personnel perform work activities at intra- and extra-hospitalary settings.

As in every profession, the benefits, risks, and results should be assessed. Thus, it is not always easy to carry out CPR on a person who is in cardiorespiratory arrest, above all when the sole objective is to prolong life regardless of the consequences generated.

In the hospital ambit, the patient, relative, or the legal representative should be informed of the patient's diagnosis, treatment, and prognosis of life, and informed consent should be obtained. But in the extra-hospitalary emergency in which the health professional encounters the fact of making a decision without taking into account the person's will, he/she is acting only in benefit of the person who needs to be given help. Therefore, what is applied is the so-called beneficence principle (seek the greatest benefit for the person and not that of others), which is contrary to the principle of autonomy (respect for the opinion of the person). In this case, there exists the option of that the patient has left instructions in what is known as a living will (known as a do-not-resuscitate order). If the principle of justice is applied to everything that can be of benefit in CPR, there should be access to the latter.

On the other hand, the international council establishes the maneuvers that should only be initiated for persons who unexpectedly experience airway obstruction and in the absence of a pulse, understanding that the Cardirespiratory arrest (CRA) should be sudden and potentially reversible and not due to the consequences of a terminal disease.

The law demands that the following be made known to the judicial authority:

- Deaths whose origin was a consequence of a violent act or that are suspected of criminality.
- Deaths in which it is not possible to adequately establish the cause of death.

This communication will be made by any person who has knowledge of the fact or by any professional who because of his/her activity has intervened. In the latter case, the judicial demands are greater. In the medical case, the following should be distinguished:

- Establish the diagnosis of death.
- Establish the signs or symptoms incompatible with life.

At the first instance, an oral communication can be made, but later this should be made in writing, by means of a legal medical document. It is not necessary to do this directly with the judicial authority, but rather through the State's security forces and bodies.

The civil and penal responsibility of the professionals involves problems of great complexity: the practice centers on the terrain of imprudence, understood as "negligent failure against persons and against property", this ending up as malpractice if it is not possible to achieve the purpose of a medical treatment or if the treatment is considered useless.

In the case of newborns, it is justified to interrupt resuscitation after 10 minutes without signs of life, despite continuous and adequate resuscitation maneuvers having been carried out.

It has been demonstrated that the prognosis of survival without disability is extremely low when there is no response within a period of >10 minutes of duration of intensive resuscitation maneuvers. There are few criteria that permit exactly predicting the effectiveness of CPR. In view of this uncertainty, all patients with cardiac arrest should be resuscitated, unless:

- The patient has a valid do-not-resuscitate order.
- The patient presents signs of irreversible death (for example, rigor mortis, decapitation, decomposition, or lividity).
- A physiological benefit cannot be expected due to the deterioration of the vital functions despite optimal treatment (for example, progressive septic shock or cardiogenic shock). Training in cardiopulmonary resuscitation exhorts the first responder/resuscitator to begin CPR. It is expected that health team personnel will perform CPR as part of their obligations.

The term judicial responsibility derives from the Latin verb *respondere,* which translates into the obligation of responding to some thing or to some person.

The concept of professional responsibility refers to the obligation of their having to respond for their acts of those who exercise a determined profession, understanding by this "the habitual performance of any paid or pro bono act or the providing of any service of each profession".

The General Health Law in Mexico, in Article 469, establishes that: the medical care professional, technician, or assistant who without just cause refuses to provide care for a person, in the case of notorious emergency, placing the person's life in danger, will be sentenced to 6 months to 5 years of prison and a fine of 5 to 128 days of the generally valid minimum salary in the economic zone involved and suspension of the exercise of their profession for up to 2 years. If harm were to be produced due to lack of intervention, the following will be imposed: definitive suspension of the exercising of the profession, at the judgment of the judicial authority. Likewise, the person can incur in civil responsibility, cited in the Federal Civil Code, which establishes the following:

Article 1910. The person who works illicitly or against the good customs causes harm to others, is obliged to make reparation for this, except if it is demonstrated that the harm was produced as a consequence of the inexcusable negligence or guilt of the victim.

The illicit deed in the obligation to respond for the harm caused when a person himself/herself makes use of dangerous mechanisms, instruments, apparatuses, or substances, independently of the guilt of the author of the deed.

Article 2104. The person who was obliged to provide a fact and who did not provide this or who did not provide this according to what has been agreed upon, will be responsible for the damages and prejudices.

The controversies aroused due to a presumed civil medical responsibility can settled in the following two ways:

1. By the jurisdictional route

Normally in these controversies, the claimant demands payment for the damages and prejudices caused by the medical care and that incurred as a result, presumably, physical harm, or even moral damage.

2. By amicable means

That is, by reason of the procedures of conciliation and arbitration taken before the National Medical Arbitration Commission for negotiation by the Commission based on the Regulations of Procedures for Attention to Medical Complaints.

Penal responsibility

Unlike civil law that specifically protects an individual's interest and that, in the case of appeal gives rise to an indemnized sanction, penal law rests on the idea of a collective value that the State should protect and that it generates for the author of a reproachable behavior a repressive sanction, as can be, among others, the crime of privation of freedom.

In this respect, Article 228 of the Federal Penal Code establishes the following: professionals, artists, or technicians and their assistants will be responsible for the crimes that are committed in the exercise of their profession, in the following terms and without the prejudice of the admonitions contained in the General Health Law of Mexico/Ley General de Salud or in other norms on the professional exercise, in the following case:

1. In addition to the sanctions fixed for crimes that are committed, whether deceitful or culpable, the suspension of 1 month to 2 years will be applied to them in the exercise of their profession or definitively in the case of relapse, and

2. They will be obliged to repair the damage caused by their own acts and those of their assistants, when the latter act according to the instructions of the former.

Article 340. Whoever finds an child abandoned at any site who is unable to care for him/herself or a wounded or disabled person or one who is threatened by any danger whatsoever, will be sentenced to 10–60 community work days if they do not immediately notify the authority or if they omit providing the necessary help when they could do this without incurring personal risk.

It is important to mention that in Mexico there is no law that protects persons who are sued for providing CPR, although there is no knowledge to date of a trained person who has provided CPR being sued and whose case proceeded to successful accusation.

Therefore, the medical practice, which is founded on the responsibility of the professional exercising medicine, demands respect for human dignity, the nobility of the human body in any situation.

Chapter 11

Use of Mechanical Devices in CPR-A

Twenty-first century science and technology has advanced acceleratedly and its being accompanied by that and the use of mechanical devices in the health sciences is truly grandiose. Technology has changed worldwide according to the needs of humans themselves, who have made such a situation possible. Human beings are innovative and at present this is conceived of as the application of technology to the solution of problems.

In the health sciences, this has permitted the facilitation of care through technology and science in real situations to improve life conditions.

The new technologies have made it possible to perform accurate diagnosis and treatments. These encompass the discovery of novel drugs and electromedical apparatuses, as well as the utilization of new techniques employed in the procedures used in the integral care of Cardiorespiratory arrest (CRA), with which attention is provided efficiently and effectively. From this focus, technology not only comprised machines or drugs, but also the clinical practice itself, which translates into efficiency, effectiveness, benefit, and excellence.

How can these technologies be used in persons presenting cardiorespiratory arrest?

In Cardiopulmonary resuscitation (CPR), the use of new technologies has made it possible to save many lives in the extra-hospitalary ambit with the use of Automatic external defibrillators (AED) and land and air transport vehicles that are duly equipped and managed by trained personal, and in the intra-hospitalary ambit with the techniques utilized to recover and strengthen the cardiorespiratory function by means of endotracheal intubation techniques, modern ventilators, but above all with the knowledge and skills of health team members.

The success of CPR is due to the prompt application of Basic cardiopulmonary resuscitation (CPR-B).

Advanced cardiopulmonary resuscitation (PCR-A)

This comprises the measures that should be applied when adequate technical and prepared-personnel means are possessed for their utilization. Their objectives are to establish adequate ventilation, reestablish cardiac activity, normalize the cardiac rhythm, and establish the hemodynamic.

Peter Safar affirms that CPR-A is the continuation of CPR-B, in addition to that in this phase II, ALS (Advanced Life Support) and other actions are performed, such as:

- The use of devices to maintain effective respiratory and circulatory function.
- The establishment of a peripheral venous route or a functional central route.
- Cardiac monitoring.
- Identification of arrhythmias.
- Use of specific drugs.
- Stabilization of the patient.

What devices are utilized in airway maintenance in CPR-A?

- Self-inflatable Artificial manual breathing unit (AMBU)/Bag valve mask (BVM).
- Oropharyngeal/nasopharyngeal cannulas.
- Equipment for endotracheal intubation.
- Defibrillator.

Bag valve mask/AMBU

The AMBU, or the self-inflatable resuscitation balloon, as it is also known, is a device that is utilized in manual ventilation. It is used to insufflate air into the airways. It is a bag connected to a unidirectional valve that in turn is connected to an assisted ventilation mask. It is placed utilizing the index fingers and the thumbs to maintain the mask fixed to the patient's face; with the other three fingers (middle, fourth, and little), the neck is extended and with the other hand, we insufflate the BVM/AMBU mask.

Oropharyngeal/nasopharyngeal cannulas

Oropharyngeal cannulas are devices that are employed to maintain the airways permeated, depressing the back part of the tongue. The placement technique includes introducing the tube with the concavity upward until the point reaches the soft palate. At this time, it rotates 180º and slides behind the tongue. In some cases, a tongue depressor and laryngoscopy can be utilized; size should be chosen according to age, taking into account the length from the upper incisors to the mandible angle. Sizes range between 4 and 10 cm in length. If the cannula used is too large or if it is placed incorrectly, it can displace the tongue backward and obstruct the airway; contrariwise, if the cannula is too short, it will not achieve the desired purpose. It is important to know that this type of cannula should not be used in conscious patients because it can induce vomiting with the risk of bronchoaspiration or laryngospasm. Other devices include the nasopharyngeal cannulas; these are employed in conscious persons because it has been evidenced that they are better tolerated by the patient. For selecting their size, it is important to know the appropriate length. There are various sizes of cannulas that range from numbers 12–36. The person who installs or places this type of cannula should have the skill and experience to do so; contrariwise, placement can produce injuries to the adenoids or to the nasal mucosa, causing hemorrhages and complicating airway permeability. The Guedel cannula is a device that is utilized frequently in emergency situations. It is made of a plastic material and its purpose it to depress the tongue and to facilitate the passage of air. For placement, it is important to choose the suitable size previously according to the patient's age; this should coincide with the distance between the buccal commissure and the angle of the mandible. For its placement, the neck should be tilted in hyperextension, opening the mouth of the victim with thumbs and index fingers of the hand that is not holding the cannula to induce it later; the concave part should be directed toward the palate, turning it progressively according to its introduction into the mouth until leaving it in its definitive position. Once installed, its correct placement should be tested. Laryngeal masks are devices that are placed on the posterior wall of the pharynx, with the purpose of sealing the region of the base of the tongue and the pharyngeal opening/aperture. This device is effective under controlled conditions and the person who installs it should have the knowledge and experience to install these masks. These are tubes that are similar to the endotracheal one that have a small mask and a circumferential balloon.

Endotracheal intubation

Endotracheal intubation is carried out when it is required to maintain assisted ventilation, or when adequate ventilation is not obtained with the BVM/AMBU mask, The procedure is considered as programmed even though it is an emergency because all of the equipment and material as been previously prepared for it to be successful, in addition to that the professional performing it must have the knowledge and skills to carry it out.

Intubation is a technique that consists of introducing a tube through the mouth (orotracheal), or on occasion through the nose (nasotracheal) of the patient, until reaching the trachea, in order to maintain the airway open and to be able to assist the patient in the breathing process. In CPR, the most commonly utilized of these is orotracheal intubation, because it is easier and faster; in CPR-A, it is the most effective method for maintaining the airway open. It has the great advantage of diminishing the risk of gastric distension and that of pulmonary aspiration. In addition, it allows the administration of some drugs during CRA in serious situations in which a venous airway has not been installed or when this is not functional. It is very useful for the aspiration of secretions.

What equipment should be prepared for endotracheal intubation?

- Complete laryngoscopy that includes:

  - Laryngoscope handle with bulb and batteries.
  - Curved or straight laryngoscope sheets.
  - Orotracheal or nasotracheal tube or catheter.
  - Stylus or guidewire.
- Fixed or portable aspiration equipment with an aspiration catheter.
- BVM/AMBU mask.
- Stethoscope.
- Lidocaine.
- Syringes.
- Surgical gloves.
- Drugs: sedatives and relaxants.

Selection of the number of the laryngoscope sheets and the size of the catheter depends on the age of the patient. The intubation technique should be carried out with the safety conferred by everything being prepared and ready to proceed. In addition to prior oxygenation of the patient, the patient's head and neck are manually immobilized to proceed; the laryngoscope is grasped in the left hand and the laryngoscope sheet is introduced at the right buccal commissure of the patient, displacing the tongue to the left in the direction of the median line. Raise the laryngoscope in a 45º direction in relation to the horizontal, without exerting pressure on the teeth or buccal tissues, visually identifying the epiglottis and then the vocal cords. With the right hand, insert the endotracheal tube into the trachea, continuing until crossing the vocal cords. The laryngoscope handle should pass from 1 to 2.5 cm within the trachea; this will place the proximal end of the tube at the level of the teeth, between 19 and 23 cm in the majority of adults. The laryngoscope handle is insufflated with 10–20 cc of air, sufficient to achieve an adequate seal. The position of the ventilation tube should be ensured by means of the tube bag valve device and observation should be made of whether there is thoracic expansion by listening at the level of the thorax. Once it has been verified that this is correct, the tube can be ensured and we can proceed to leave this perfectly fixed.

Defibrillator

An implantable Automatic external defibrillator (AED) is a device that is utilized in CPR-A and that possesses a function with which it can detect an abnormal cardiac rhythm and revert it automatically, in a previously programmed manner, by means of anti-tachycardia stimulation or by electric shocks.

Defibrillation (DF) is the treatment-of-choice in the case of the Ventricular fibrillation (VF) of Ventricular tachycardia without a pulse (VTSP) and in Cardioversion (CV). It is a treatment that is commonly used in arrhythmias with hemodynamic repercussion. DF and CV are procedures that consist of applying a low-voltage electric shock, which causes the simultaneous depolarization of all of the myocardial cells. In DF, the discharge is sudden, while in CV, the discharge is synchronized, which allows that from the performance of DF or of CV, normal cardiac activity can be recovered and it renders the heartbeats spontaneous and coordinated once more.

The defibrillator is an electrical energy condenser that is composed of some contact paddles and an electrode interface that is the conductor means whose function it is to permit the passage of the electrical current through the skin. Similar to previous devices, it is indispensible that the person utilizing the device knows the functioning of the DF and possesses the knowledge, experience, and skill to perform the technique. Additionally, because it is habitually required in emergency situations in which life is in danger, it is important to know that the paddle size is chosen according to the patient's age and the size of the patient's thorax.

What equipment should be prepared for defibrillation in CPR-A?

The equipment that is utilized for electrical DF or CV is the following:

- Defibrillator: energy condenser that is basically the monitor.
- Paddles: of which there are two different sizes.
- Electrode interface: allows the passage of current through the skin after prior impregnation with gel or conductive paste.

How is defibrillation performed in CPR- A?

To initiate DF, the following is performed:

- Lubricate the paddles of the defibrillator with conductive paste and care should be taken to avoid contact between the two paddles.
- Put the command on "asynchronic" in the case of DF.
- Charge DF at 2–4 J/kg or CV at 0.5–1 J/kg.
- Place the pressured paddles against the thorax, one in the left-side infraclavicular region and the other at the left-side apex.
- Prior to initiating the discharge, caution should be taken that those who are around the patient be separated from the patient.
- Again verify that the patient does indeed have a cardiac problem.
- Immediately and simultaneously press the buttons of both paddles, effect the discharge, and test whether the shock has been produced by verifying the monitor (which is found previously installed in the patient) and that there is movement in the isoelectric line of the monitor, and verify whether the Electrocardiographic (EEG) rhythm has been modified.

This is a procedure that is carried out rapidly and with equipment synchrony for the treatment of the DF. In addition, there should be agreements regarding the dynamic of participation in each hospital area in which the procedure is conducted.

Continuation of the treatment in the patient who has reverted the CRA is continued in phase III, which is that of intensive life support and that is based for practical purposes on correcting the cause of the CRA. In this phase, the intervention of treatment in the Intensive Care Unit (ICU) and of the participation of specialized personnel considers that the treatment of the CRA is an intensive and continuous process from the moment of identifying the CRA until the time that it is reverted.

In intensive life support, post-resuscitation care will have as its objective the optimization of the function of the diverse organ systems that can be primarily or secondarily compromised to hypoxia, especially post-anoxic encephalopathy. Thus, the care will comprise the following:

- Assessment of the patient's recovery and of the cause that gave rise to the CRA.
- Control of the diverse organs and systems, with optimization of the treatment of these.

Breathing support techniques comprise the following: mechanically controlled breathing and assisted mechanical breathing. In the former, the ventilator provides the volume of the current that is previously determined, independently of the patient's ventilatory impulses; in the latter, the inspiratory valve functions as a demand valve and the patient is able to trigger a breath in order to make an inspiratory effort; despite that the patient triggers the ventilator, this is not a spontaneous breath because the ventilator will apply the programmed current volume.

The patient who has recovered from Cardiac arrest (CA) is at risk for again incurring CA in the subsequent hours; thus, the patient should be managed in an ICU. Reactions can be different in each person. Bearing in mind that each human being is unique and unrepeatable and that each has different response patterns, reactions can range from the person who recovers consciousness, breathes, and presents a stable hemodynamic, to the individual who persists in being comatose, does not breathe, and maintains an unstable hemodynamic.

On concluding this chapter, it is important to consider that humans acts indistinctly over time, thinking of the past, planning the future, and never truly living and enjoying the present. We have only one life and we must live it, because we never know when it will come to an end.

Chapter 12

The Importance of the Administration of Drugs Utilized in CPR-A

Advances in the clinical sciences are under constant change. Pharmacological therapeutics orders the information necessary to know at what exact moment the utilization is necessary of treatments and drug use, of the activities directly involving the personnel who constantly have the responsibility of administering drugs and observing their effects.

Cardiorespiratory arrest (CRA) is the most critical emergency that has presented in the history of mankind in the extra- and intra-hospitalary ambit because when it is not identified in timely fashion, it has fatal consequences. Thus, it is important for persons, found or not in the health ambit, to be prepared and to know what to do immediately and how to act in the face of this emergency. Therefore, the lives of many persons could be saved.

Basic cardiopulmonary resuscitation (CPR-B) should be given immediately after identifying CRA. It is important to remember that the time between the arrest and the resuscitation, as well as the time that it takes to reestablish the cardiac rhythm that allows reestablishing organic perfusion, is transcendental for the final prognosis.

In the hospital areas, health professionals form an important part of the multidisciplinary team; those confronting emergency situations require technical, scientific, and ethical knowledge. In the majority of times, the therapeutic success of Advanced cardiopulmonary resuscitation (CPR-A) rests upon on the speed with which the drugs are administered by one of the team members, although more often that not this responsibility falls to the nursing professionals. Those in charge of this task should follow the therapeutic indications in urgent and in emergency situations. Thus, possessing broad and scientific preparation is of vital importance in this respect.

The circumstances of action are diverse in the hospital ambit; one of these is the emergency care of a patient with CRA, in that the event merits offering an immediate and professional response that permits them to resolve the event that presents in the most ideal manner, by means of an accurate participation and one accompanied by scientific knowledge, due to that the activities involved in drug administration and their direct contact with the sick individual, the importance should be considered of possessing the know-how and having at hand the action, doses, and administration routes, as well as the adverse effects that each drug has in relation to the event requiring its utilization (this revolves around taking the actions the actions that should be borne in mind with respect to normativity in the administration of the drugs).

In the previous chapters, we have explained that related with basic CPR. In this chapter, some aspects will be approached that are related with the use of drugs in the second phase of CPR-A. According to the classification of Peter Safar, for CPAR-A to be viable, the first phase of CPR-B? must have been carried out effectively by trained persons.

In CPR-A, a trained person should guide the actions and is directly responsible for verifying the following:

- That the CPR-B has been correct.
- That there is an installation and maintenance of a permeable and functional airway.
- That the pharmacological is correct.
- That endotracheal intubation is performed.
- That Defibrillation is carried out.
- That the decision is made concerning the moment at which CPR is finalized.

In CPR-A, the installation and maintenance of a permeable and functional airway is something fundamental that will coadjuvate in having the best possibilities of survival, and this is related with the speed with which it is carried out, in addition to maintaining the airway, strengthening the circulation, Defibrillation (DF), drug administration, and obtaining a venous route for the perfusion of these. There are various ways of installing a venous route, which depends on the general conditions in which the patient is found. In the case of CPR, there are the following:

- Peripheral venous route.
- Central venous route.
- Endotracheal route.

Each of these has its own specifications and here are the following:

The peripheral venous route should preferentially be installed at the level of, or above the level of, the diaphragm; it is recommended that this be in the antecubital vein, which is safer and faster to obtain. In addition to having the advantage of being able to be catheterized, it is not necessary to delay the CPR maneuvers. When a person with this skill is available, a long catheter can be inserted into this vein. When the drug is administered by peripheral route in a patient with CRA, this drug takes somewhat longer to enter the central circulation, which is much delayed; thus, it is recommended that a drug always be administered in diluted form so that its arrival in the bloodstream will be faster. In addition, it is recommended that the limb in which the venous route is installed be raised so that the drug can reach it more rapidly.

The central venous route possesses the great advantage of the *rapidity* with which the drugs reach the central circulation and are distributed to the vital organs. But the disadvantage is that only personnel with the knowledge and the skill can install it in the least possible amount of time. The venous accesses are in the internal jugular vein and in the subclavial vein. The choice of one or the other depends on the practice of the person who is to carry this out.

The endotracheal route is utilized for drug administration when, due to the seriousness of the patient's state, it is not possible to install either of the previous two if the patient has already been intubated. Although it is important to remember that doses vary in relation to those administered by venous route, it is noteworthy that this route is only utilized in cases that involve strictly emergency scenarios.

There are other routes for drug administration during CPR that are less frequently employed less frequently in current practice during CPR; this is due to the side effects and the complications with which their utilization is consequently accompanied. These other routes comprise the intra-osseous and the intra-cardiac routes.

The venous routes are essential during CPR-A maneuvers. Thus, the maintenance and permeability of these are very important, as is their functionality.

With respect to the drugs, these should be localized in the first drawer of the RC; the order of these can be subject to change, according to the structure of the RC and to the hospital routine (Table 10-1).

On the other hand, it is important to consider that the drugs utilized in CPR-A should be localized in a specific place, such as the **Red Cart (RC)**, which is a necessary piece of equipment that is required mainly in the emergency room, but that is also highly important in other areas of the hospital. This cart should have the equipment, drugs, and specialized materials for resolving health problems meriting urgent attention. The RC is utilized in urgent situations and when life is at risk, whether due to a sudden disease manifestation or to trauma.

With respect to the drugs, these should be localized in the first drawer of the RC; the order of these can be subject to change, according to the structure of the RC and to the hospital routine.

It is important to remember that the first drawer of the RC has 265 compartments and that each drug is ordered and accommodated in the previously mentioned order, observing the importance of the first three, which are utilized in CPR.

As noted previously, the rapidity with which each and every CPR maneuver is carried out in all of its phases will transfer into the success obtained in these situations that comprise a true emergency in patient care.

Drug	Amounts
1. Adrenaline	10
2. Atrophin	10
3. Sodium bicarbonate	4
4. Aminofilin	20
5. Potassium chloride	4
6. Dexamethazone	8
7. Diazepam	4
8. Diphenylhydantoin (DPH)	4
9. Diphenydramine	2

Drug	Amounts
10. Diazoxide	4
11. Digoxin	5
12. Dobutamine	4
13. Dopamine	4
14. Flunitrazepam	4
15. Furosemide	6
16. Calcium gluconate	4
17. Glucose at 50%	4
18. Hydrocortisone	5
19. Isoproterenol	1
20. Methylprednisolone	5
21. Sodium nitroprussiate	2
22. Magnesium sulfate	10
23. Verapamil	4
24. Simple xylocaine at 1%	1
25. Simple xylocaine at 2%	1
26. Xylocaine at 10% in spray	1

Table 10-1. Drugs included in the **Red Cart (RC)**

References

American Heart Association. (2006). Soporte Vital Basico para Personal del Equipo de Salud. Prous Science

American Heart Association. 2010 CPR and ECC Guidelines.www.heart.org/ cpr

Brunner Sholtis, L. (1998). *Enfermeria Medico Quirurgica* (Vol. 2). Interamericana.

Chapleau, W. (2007). *Primer Interviniente en Emergencias: Marcando la Diferencia.* Madrid, España: Elsevier España, S.A.

Cisneros, F.J. Rivas. (2006) paro cardíaco y embarazo, vol. 29.

Código Penal Federal. México 2012.

Comision inter institucional de enfermería. (2011). *Codigo de etica para enfermeras y enfermeros de méxico.* D.F., México: Subsecretaria de inovación y calidad.

Davis, A., & Tschundin, V. (2009). Etica en enfermeria, conceptos fundamentales en su enseñanza.

DeCherney, A., Nathan, L., Goodwin, M., & Laufer, N. (2007). *Diagnostico y tratamiento gineco obstétrico* (9 ed.). (I. d. Monteón Batalla, Trad.) D.F., México: Manual Moderno S.A. de C.V.

Department of Health, Welsh Office, Scottish Office Department oh Health and Social Services, Northern Ireland Why mothers die. Report on confidential.

Emad Atta, MDa, y Michael Gardner, MD, MPHb Reanimación cardiopulmonar en el embarazo,* A Department of Obstetrics and Gynecology, Medical College of Georgia,1120 15th Street, Augusta, GA 30912, USA Division of Maternal Fetal Medicine, Department of Gynecology and Obstetrics,Emory University School of Medicine, 69 Jesse Hill Jr. Drive SE,Atlanta, GA 30303, USA

Guías clínicas obstétricas y ginecológicas de Norteamérica, (2009)

Johnson MD, Luppi CJ, Over DC Cardiopulmonary resuscitation. In Gambling DR Douglas MJ, editors. Obstetric Anesthesia and uncommon disorders. Philadelphia: WB Saunders:1998.p51-74

Kerr Mg The mechanical effects of the gravid uterus in late pregnancy.J Obstet Gynaecol Br Commw 1965; 72513-29

Ley General de Salud. México 2012.

Morris S, Stacey M. Resuscitation in pregnancy. BMJ 2003; 327.

Ortega Deballón, I. M, "Ética y responsabilidad legal del personal sanitario en las urgencias, emergencias y catástrofes". En formación continuada de Urgencias y emergencias sanitarias. Ed Formación Alcalá. Jaén.2002.

Ortega Deballón. I. M, "Aspectos éticos-legales en las emergencias Extrahospitalarias". Artículo de la revista Metas de Enfermería 2002, Numero 48, paginas 26-30.

Peralta Rodríguez Narciso Manual de Soporte Básico Avanzado 4ª Edición editorial Elsevier Mason 2007

Poole JH, Long J Maternal mortality-a review of current treds. Crit Care Nurs Clin North Am 2004;16:227-30

Rodríguez Palomares Consuelo. Farmacología para enfermeras Mc Graw Hill Interamericana editores S.A.de C.V, 2007

Rovira Gil, E; López González, A; García Fernández, C. "Ética y reanimación cardiopulmonar: visión actualizada. Artículo de la revista de enfermería 1999; Número 9: Pagina 39-42.

Whitty JE. Maternal Cardiac arrest in pregnancy. Clin Obstet Gynecol 2002;45:377-92

www.slideshare.net/.../reanimacin-cardio-pulmonar-en-embarazo consultado en diciembre 2012

Additional references

Feyto Grande, L. (2009). *Etica y enfermeria.*

Lemone, P. (2009). Enfermeria medico quirurgica, pensamiento critico en la atención del paciente (4 ed.). Pearson Prentice Hall.

Morales Gonzales, J. A. (2011). *Etica, bioetica y conocimiento del hombre.* D.F., México.

Morillo, J. (2007). *Manual de Enfermeria: Asistencia Prehospitalaria Urgente.* Madrid, España: Elsevier España, S.A.

Peralta Rodriguez, N. (2007). *Manual de soporte basico avanzado* (4 ed.). Elsevier Mason.

Real Academia de la Lengua Española. (s.f.). *Real Academia Española.* Recuperado el 1 de abril de 2011, de http://www.rae.es

Rodriguez Lozano, V. (1998). *Ética.* Pearson educación.

Rodriguez Palomares, C. (2007). *farmacologia para enfermeras.* Mc. Graw Hill Interamericana editores S.A. de C.V.

T., D. Cuidados de la enfermera reanimación. Taray-Masson.